The Teen Eating Manifesto:

The Ten Essential Steps to Losing Weight, Looking Great and Getting Healthy

Lisa Stollman, MA, RD, CDE, CDN

Published by Nirvana Press

No part of this publication may be reproduced, stored in a retrieval system, or transmitted in any form or by any means, electronic, mechanical, photocopying, recording, scanning, or otherwise, except as permitted under Section 107 of the 1976 United States Copyright Act, without either the prior written permission of the Publisher. Requests to the Publisher for permission should be addressed to:
Nirvana Press, 240 Main Street, P.O. Box 667, Northport, NY 11768,
www.nirvanapressny.com

Stollman, Lisa
The Teen Eating Eating Manifesto: The Ten Essential Steps for Losing Weight, Looking Great and Getting Healthy

ISBN 978-0-9852296-0-3 (pbk.)

Printed in the United States of America

Published by Nirvana Press, Northport, New York.

Dedication

This book is dedicated to my sons' Sam and Max, who are my pride and joy; my soul mate, Eric, who has nourished me with his love and sheer brilliance for almost thirty years, my Puli pup, Laszlo, who brings an abundance of joy to our household; my lifelong pal, Susan Kroll, who I love and adore. And, last but not least, my mother, who instilled in me her passion for healthy and delicious food. I know she is smiling from up above.

Acknowledgements

Many thanks are owed to all of the people who helped transform my ideas into this book. To my fabulous interns, Lindsay Moyer and Lauren Ann Zimmerman, who are both nutrition graduate students and published writers themselves. You are the BEST! I'm sure you will both go very far in your nutrition careers. To my highly-esteemed colleagues from the Pediatric Subunit of the Weight Management Practice Group of The Academy of Nutrition and Dietetics: Christine Clarahan, RD, Barbie Cervino, MS, RD, CDE, CDN, Yvette Gideon, RD, LDN, Ciara Halpin, RD, Blanche Keir, RD and Debbie Wong, MPH, RD. Thank you so much for your editing skills and professional advice. Each of you gave me your time and I so appreciate it. To my pediatric colleagues, Dr. Ken Prushik, MD, Dr. Paul Shineman, MD, Dr. Kathrynne Yland, MD, Dr. Sharon Inkeles, MD and Dr. Sharyn Solish, MD: thank you so much for taking the time to review my manuscript and give your expert feedback. To my wonderful friend, Ann Silver, MS, RD, CDE, CDN for your valuable comments and edits. And, last but not least, my amazing husband, Eric Smouha, MD who also took time from his busy schedule to review my book and provide his terrific insight.

Introduction

Why did I write this book? For over twenty-five years I have worked as a Registered Dietitian and Nutritionist helping people of all ages, from young children to those over eighty, lose weight and improve their health. I have found what works–and what doesn't--for eating well and having a healthy weight. As a teen, I also had issues with my weight. Over time (majoring in nutrition was a huge help!) I learned how to eat right and have a healthy lifestyle. It would have been **so** much easier for me if I had a helpful book **then** that taught me how to eat healthy and manage my weight. You shouldn't have to have a college degree in nutrition to know how to eat well! This is why I saw the profound need to compile my knowledge and experience into this book so you can learn how to apply these healthy eating and lifestyle skills into your daily routine. Believe me, I know firsthand that it's wise to learn good eating skills when you are young as it will be so much easier to make healthy eating a regular part of your life and avoid many of the chronic diseases, such as heart disease, diabetes and various types of cancer, that are seen in epidemic proportions today.

I'll share my secret with you.

Having a healthy meal routine and a commitment to regular exercise will help you get to your desired weight goal. If you continue to eat well and exercise, you can stay at this weight goal for life. You can make **two smart moves** for yourself **now**:

Learn how to make (1) **healthy eating** combined with (2) **regular exercise** part of your lifestyle.

These two valuable skills will benefit you for many years to come. You'll enjoy a healthier weight; you'll also look and feel great, plus you'll reduce your risk for many long-term health problems, such as Type 2 diabetes and heart disease.

Maybe you've tried to lose weight in the past but didn't get very far. Perhaps you lost ten to twenty pounds by following a diet, only to quickly regain the weight back. That's OK! I'm here to help you figure out how to make this time **different**. You'll decide how to make changes in the foods you eat and in your daily life that you can stick to for good. These changes will soon become habits (it takes about 30 days for a **change** to become a habit) that you keep up—even after you get to your goal weight.

Yes, it sounds simple! But these are your keys to losing weight and keeping it off for a lifetime.

Before we get started, I want to give you one piece of advice. *Fad diets don't work.* Many people—teens and adults included—go on one fad diet after another, losing weight only to regain it back (and many times gaining back a lot more than they lost!). They are quick fix, short-term plans that promise miraculous results, such as losing ten pounds in one week (!) and don't teach you how to eat well in the real world. Spending your life going from one hopeless and (boring!) fad diet to the next is not a road you need to travel. If you've made it this far, you might have guessed why: Fad diets don't help you find a way to eat and live sensibly.

Fad diets start a vicious cycle that is hard to break. Instead, I want to help you create a real-life plan that works for *you* and makes you feel good. Having the knowledge to eat well and make exercise a part of your life will help you be confident, lose weight, and keep it off for good. And the outcome for you will be a healthy and happy life without the physical struggles and illnesses a weight problem can bring. Feeling better and being healthier go hand in hand when you eat well. Devoting yourself to a lifestyle that includes exercise and eating a healthy diet with moderate portions is the best method to lose weight and to keep it off. Most people, who make the change from a typical low fiber/high-fat diet and sedentary lifestyle to one that includes a diet rich in healthy high fiber/moderate-fat coupled with regular exercise, will slowly and safely lose weight.

In this book you will explore the ten steps to eating well, losing weight, looking great and improving your health. You will also find awesome strategies for eating healthy at parties, on vacation, in restaurants, etc. as well as a treasure trove of tools including a sample meal plan, a one-week menu, tasty recipes and a healthy shopping list. You can start the book in any order you choose, but you might find it most helpful to start with Step 1. Develop a Meal Routine, which I believe is the most important step. You're starting a journey to figure out a lifelong *eating plan*, not a gimmicky, fad "diet." Learning how to implement a meal routine will get you off to a great start!

Before I continue I just want to quickly introduce myself. I was born and grew up in Detroit (also known as The Motor City and — which I affectionately call—Motown!). Cooking and healthy eating have been passions of mine since I was about fifteen years old. After high school I moved to the east coast to study nutrition at New York University. I loved the program at NYU so much that after I obtained my B.S. in Foods and Nutrition, I stayed on for graduate school and received my M.A. in Clinical Nutrition. And I've never looked back! I truly love what I do–helping teens and adults improve their lives by eating healthy and managing their weight.

Congrats on making this important health choice for yourself! Taking the time now to develop the important skills of healthy eating and weight management will improve the quality of your life for many years to come. ***Good luck!***

Table of Contents

Getting Started with the Ten Steps

Are You Ready To Eat Healthier and Lose Weight?

When you decide you want to lose weight, **you** should be prepared to make a commitment to yourself. You need to be ready to modify your eating habits and start a regular exercise program. Unless your extra weight is causing health problems now, **you** should make the decision to lose weight and improve your health *for yourself.* Of course, losing any extra pounds will help you be healthier and feel better, now and in the future. But you need to be sure that **you** are ready.

What do I mean? Just because your friends are losing weight or your parents have been on your case, don't feel that you need to lose weight *now*. When you are ready, you will know. And you will do it for **yourself** because you want to. Anyone can lose weight, but the key is making the weight loss sustainable. When I say "sustainable," I mean keeping the weight off. Otherwise you may suffer through a lifetime of going on and off diets—otherwise known as "yo-yo dieting." You can become very frustrated if losing weight is a constant in your life.

Learning how to lose and maintain weight is a powerful skill. We all know that there is no fairy dust that can be sprinkled to help you magically lose weight. But it doesn't have to be difficult and you shouldn't feel deprived. I have worked with many people who have been burdened with extra weight for many years. These individuals have shown me that by making nutritious food choices and having a regular exercise program, you too, can enjoy a healthy weight for life.

Do you want to lose weight to look better in your clothes, or do you want to be more physically fit? Do you want to lose the extra pounds so you can try out for a school sports team? Maybe you want to lose weight because your mother or father has diabetes and you want to lower your risk. Having a goal in mind as you start your weight loss journey will help you stay focused and get you to your desired weight. And always, no matter what, love yourself! Whether you find that eating healthy and exercising come easy to you or you find it a struggle to get and stay on track, if you love yourself, it will make if that much easier to succeed. Don't get down on yourself if you encounter hurdles. We all encounter hurdles, whether it's weight, school, work or relationships. If you love yourself, and by that I mean truly liking yourself as a person, you will find the way to get through these obstacles and do what is best for you!

Let's get started with your goal and the ten steps to help you lose weight, look great, and get healthy!

The Ten Essential Steps

Step 1. Get a Meal Routine

Step 2. Practice Mindful Eating

Step 3. Stay on Track with Self-Monitoring

Step 4. Exercise: Move It to Lose It!

Step 5. Cut Down on Sugar (aka Junk Food)

Step 6. Don' Drink Your Calories

Step 7. Fill Up on Fiber

Step 8. Eat Less Fat and Choose Them Wisely

Step 9. Read Food Labels

Step 10. Get Sufficient Sleep

Step 1. Get a Meal Routine

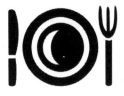

Having a meal routine is the basis for reaching, as well as maintaining, a healthy weight.

What is a meal routine?

A meal routine is a daily schedule for your meals and snacks. It means you eat breakfast, lunch, and dinner at approximately the same times each day. It also may mean you typically grab a snack between lunch and dinner. And maybe after dinner, too! With this sort of routine you get to know **the types and amounts of food that work for you** at each meal or snack. This "eating schedule" is just like your daily routine of classes throughout the school day. Having a meal routine will keep you on track so you don't miss a meal and get overly hungry. You might not realize it but when you are very hungry you tend to eat too much when you do finally take the time to eat. This can sabotage your efforts to lose weight and can, in fact, add on more pounds.

Try to visualize this scenario. You probably have experienced the feeling of excessive hunger when you didn't have time to eat lunch and now it's 2:00 PM. Your last meal was breakfast at 7:00 AM. It's now been seven hours since your last meal and you feel lightheaded, a little shaky, maybe even slightly nauseous and are starving. This is not a healthy situation to be in! Keeping a couple of healthy granola bars (such as a Kashi TLC or Kind Bar) or a peanut butter sandwich in your backpack to eat at lunch time would have helped you avoid this.

Why do you need a meal routine?

Having designated times for meals and snacks keeps your body fueled so you have the energy to accomplish what you need to do throughout the day. **Bottom line: if you have a meal routine, you will learn how to plan your eating into your daily life.**
And there's an added benefit of regular eating:

A meal routine will help you reach your desired weight goal!

You most likely have friends who are either trying to lose weight now or have in the past. Some of them may only eat one or two meals per day. And some of your friends may go without eating for a day, to speed up their weight loss, and feel fine. But neither of these scenarios are healthy or sustainable. They won't result in losing weight and staying at a healthy weight. In fact recent studies show that teens who regularly "diet" tend to be heavier in the long run. Eating well is the way to go–"dieting" is not!

So how do you lose weight and make it last? **Find a meal routine that fits your lifestyle but also has you eating about every three to five hours.** You'll need to choose a regularly scheduled time for breakfast, lunch, and dinner (Note: weekend and vacation meal times may differ if you sleep late. Simply adjust your meal routine to meet your schedule). You'll stay on track and you *won't* miss a meal, get too hungry, and overeat. Also one more important thing to cover: **Try to eat with your family a least three times per week.** Studies show that teens that eat with their families tend to eat better. Even one of my sons tells me that he eats less fruit and vegetables when he is away at college than when he's eating at home with our family! But he's working on doing better! Until you go away to college or out on your own, try to have breakfast, lunch or dinner at least three times a week with your family.

Before we go on I just want to say three very important words: **Don't skip breakfast!** Breakfast is truly the most important meal of your day. Skipping breakfast seems like a quick fix to lose weight. But in the long-term, it's actually the opposite. After sleeping for eight hours you wake up and your body's gas tank is on empty. If you don't eat, your metabolism will slow down like a car without gas. Eating breakfast kick starts your metabolism, and helps your body burn more calories, which helps you lose weight. If you want to lose weight and/or maintain a healthy weight, **start every day with breakfast**!

So what would a daily meal routine look like?

Here's a typical daily meal routine. Yours may look like this one, or not, depending on your calorie needs and how much you exercise. On weekends and during vacations you may sleep later so you can modify your meal schedule as needed. Then you'll be well on your way to starting a healthy meal routine!

Sample Meal Routine

For many teens a meal routine looks like this:

7 AM:	Breakfast
12 PM:	Lunch
3 or 4 PM:	Snack (optional)
6 PM:	Dinner
9 PM:	Snack (optional)

What is a healthy meal?

It helps to picture it. In June 2011 the U.S. government unveiled the new mealplanning icon: MyPlate (www.myplate.gov).

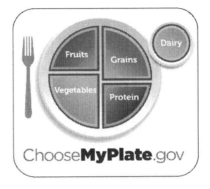

It's a great tool to visualize how much of each food group to put on your plate. Following the MyPlate approach is an easy way to plan a meal with a good variety of nutrients. As you can see from the MyPlate icon, 1/2 of your plate should be non-starchy vegetables (such as broccoli, cauliflower or carrots) and/or fruit, 1/4 should be a whole grain (such as whole grain bread, brown rice or quinoa) or starchy-vegetable (such as baked potato or butternut squash) and 1/4 should be a protein. Meal and snack ideas are provided in the sample meal plan on Page 14 and in Part 3. Tools of the Trade.

Healthy Diet Basics for Planning Your Meal Routine

So, you've mastered the meal routine. You know *when* to eat. But *what* exactly should you eat? Here's when it helps to review some basics of a healthy diet. A healthy, well-balanced diet should consist of three meals per day and, if needed, one to two snacks. Whether you need snacks depends on your calorie needs and how much you exercise. Some people feel well with eating only three times per day, and that's fine. You may find that on some days you are hungry between meals and need a snack. Maybe you had a smaller breakfast or lunch, or you exercised. You need to see what works for you.

Here's the goal. Make sure your meals contain a healthy balance of protein and carbohydrate so you will be satisfied for several hours. When you don't have a balance of this healthy duo, you may find that you get hungry much sooner. **So in what foods do you find these important nutrients?** Healthy proteins include fish, beans, chicken, nuts, tofu, seitan, tempeh, lean meat, eggs, milk, soymilk, yogurt and low fat cheese. As for carbohydrates, complex carbohydrates (also known as plant-foods), are the most nutritious. These healthy carbohydrates, in addition to being nutrient powerhouses, are rich sources of dietary fiber which will fill you up **faster** and keep you full **longer**. Complex carbohydrates include: fruits, vegetables (non-starchy and starchy), whole grains (such as quinoa, brown rice and buckwheat, breads and cereals) plus beans. If you don't have a healthy balance at each meal, you may feel hungry soon after eating and eat more often. You may also find that having a small amount of fat (such as a tablespoon of nuts or nut butter or a couple slices of avocado or a teaspoon of olive oil) at your meals and/or snack will tide you over even longer.

> **This is an easy test:** It should take three to five hours after you eat a meal to feel hungry again (if you feel hungry 2 1/2 hours or less after eating, you should look at the overall combination of your meal or snack—maybe you need more protein or fiber or a little fat at your meal or snack).

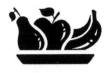

Many teens find they need a snack after school. If you need a snack, you can plan that into your day, too. First, it's wise to start off the snack with a large glass of water. Why? Because the sensation of thirst can feel the same as hunger. The result? You may often feel thirsty but confuse it with hunger and eat. If you aren't hungry after you drink the water, then go do something else. If you are truly hungry, you will know. Some people find they also need a snack after dinner, especially if they stay up late for a sport or to study. If you do, plan your snack and try to keep the calories to 200 or less. A healthy granola bar and/or a serving of fruit or a cup of whole grain cereal and skim milk may just do the trick.

What's up With Calories?

Food gives you the energy (or "fuel") to help you function throughout the day. The food you eat contains **calories** which are made up of proteins, fats and carbohydrates. Vitamins, minerals and water are also essential for good health but they don't provide calories. In case you didn't know, **calories are the energy source for our bodies.** Calories are our fuel.

Each food provides us with a different amount of calories or energy. The calories in each food is the amount of stored energy in that particular food. The number of calories you need per day is dependent upon a variety of factors including your gender, age, height, present weight and activity level.

In a nutshell, the foods you eat keep your body moving, breathing and in good health. When you don't make good food choices, you may find that you have less energy or feel irritable. You could also be more susceptible to getting sick and may find it hard to concentrate in school.

Choose Whole Foods

A smart way to make good choices is to choose a diet based on **whole foods**. Whole foods are foods that are processed and refined *as little as possible*. Whole foods typically do not contain added ingredients, such as artificial colorings and flavorings, added sugars and salt. "Whole foods" are whole grains (which includes breads, cereals and pasta), fresh fruits, starchy and non-starchy vegetables, dairy (milk, cheese and yogurt) and non-dairy alternatives such as calcium-fortified soy and almond milk, protein foods (including chicken, fish, tofu and beans) and natural oils and fats, such as avocado, peanut butter and olive oil. What's *not* a "whole food?" Chips, candy, cookies, sodas and many other packaged snack foods that contain a lot of sugar and refined grains, such as white bread. These are all known as **refined carbohydrates**. Minimize your intake of these processed, low fiber, nutrient-poor foods and you will be ahead of the game!

Here's a list of healthy whole foods:

Healthy Whole Food Choices for Your Daily Meal Routine

Dairy/Non-dairy alternatives–Skim milk, soy and almond milk, yogurt, soy yogurt

Fruit– All fresh, frozen and dried fruits

Non-starchy vegetables–broccoli, cauliflower, spinach, carrots, asparagus, artichokes, eggplant, zucchini, Brussels sprouts, kale, tomatoes, cucumbers, lettuce, Bok Choy, beets, string beans, mushrooms, okra, cabbage

Starchy vegetables–corn, peas, potatoes, butternut squash, beans, pumpkin,

Whole Grains–whole grain and multigrain cereals and breads, whole wheat, barley, millet, quinoa (pronounced "keen-wa") brown rice, whole grain pasta, buckwheat, farro, amaranth, teff.

Protein–fish, tofu, chicken, lean meat, nuts and nut butter, seeds, beans, seitan (wheat gluten), tempeh, eggs, cheese

Fats–olive oil, olives, nuts, nut butter, avocado, canola oil

Your daily meal routine may look similar to this:

Breakfast: before school between 6:00 and 7:30 AM/weekends 8:00 to 11:00 AM
1 cup high fiber cereal or granola bar or 2 waffles or 2 slices whole wheat toast or English muffin
1 cup skim or 1% milk or calcium-fortified soy milk or almond milk
1 oz. low fat cheese or 1 egg or 10 nuts or ½ cup 1% cottage cheese
1 serving fruit
tea or coffee (optional)

Lunch: between 12:00 PM and 2:00 PM
3 oz. lean protein (fish or poultry) or 8 oz. tofu or 2 tbsp. peanut butter or 4 tbsp hummus
2 slices whole grain bread or 1 sandwich thin or 1 cup beans
1 tsp olive oil or 1 ounce (3 slices) avocado
salad or raw or cooked vegetables
water

Snack: around 3:00 PM to 4:00 PM (if hungry)
1 serving fruit
1 oz. cheese or 10 nuts or 1 cup nonfat plain yogurt or smoothie (see smoothie recipes in Part 3. Tools of the Trade) or 1 can vegetable soup or 1 cup low sugar cereal (ie., Cheerios or Barbara's Cinnamon Puffins) + 1 cup skim or soy milk

Dinner: between 6:00 PM and 7:30 PM
3 oz. chicken, fish, lean meat or 8 oz. tofu or veggie burger
salad
unlimited non-starchy vegetables
2 tbsp. low fat salad dressing or 1 tbsp olive oil/vinegar/lemon
2/3 cup pasta or 1 small potato or 1 cup beans or 2 slices whole grain bread

Snack: around 9:00 pm (if hungry)
1 serving fruit and/or 1 cup nonfat yogurt or 1 cheese stick or 1 granola bar

Make sure that you have a food scale plus measuring cups and spoons on hand (these are available in the grocery store) so you can be sure that you are eating the right portion size.

Now that you know what a meal routine is, read **Step 2. Practice Mindful Eating** to become more aware of **what and how** you eat.

Step 2.   Practice Mindful Eating

Are you a Mindful Eater?

So now you've gotten into a meal routine that helps you decide *when* to eat and *what* to eat. The next step: Let's take a closer look at *how* you eat.

How quickly do you eat? When you go out with friends, are you the first to finish your meal? Do you take a second bite before you've finished your first? How many times do you chew your food before you swallow?

Where do you eat? At the table, standing at the refrigerator, watching television or in your car? (Hopefully you're not driving at the same time!)

Do you eat when you're hungry? Sometimes you may eat for other reasons—being happy, upset, lonely or bored, for example. I've seen the answers to these questions have a big impact on many teens' weight loss. One of my clients, John, a 17-year old athlete, was always the first one done with his meal, whether he was home eating with his family or out with his friends. If he was eating with his parents, and they were not yet finished with dinner, he would fill up his plate again even though he felt full. When he was out with his friends, which occurred at least twice a week, he was always the first one done with his meal. Because they were still enjoying the food on their plates, he would ask the waitress to bring him a dessert so he could keep his chums company. Over the course of his senior year he gained almost twenty pounds. By teaching John to **slow** down his eating and be more mindful when he feels full, he was able to lose the extra weight. Let's take a closer look at your habits so you can find ways to eat mindfully, too.

Practice the Simple Steps to Eating Slowly

Learning to **slow** down your eating can help you eat less. You should find that you fill up sooner and may even leave some food on your plate.

What does eating slowly look like? At your next meal, try these five steps:

1. Take a small bite.

2. Put the fork, sandwich, or slice of pizza back on the plate.

3. Chew your food twenty times while you count **slowly** to twenty.

4. Swallow.

5. Now pick up the fork or sandwich, take the next small bite and continue on as above.

Here's what happens next.

When you feel the first sensation of fullness, your stomach is telling your brain you've eaten enough. You may feel a slight tightness in your stomach. That's the time to stop. About 15 minutes later you should feel even fuller. If you keep eating after that first feeling of fullness, you'll probably feel stuffed soon. Of course, continuing to eat can make it harder to lose weight because you're getting more calories. But it can also lead to indigestion, bloating, gas, and nausea. Whether you're on a date, sitting in class, or hanging out with friends, you probably don't want to be overly full and sluggish. You want to feel your best!

So slow down your eating and stop when you feel the first feeling of getting full—and you'll speed up your weight loss.

For those who don't know when they are full because they don't feel the "fullness sensation," it is wise to stop eating after you finish your first plate of food and do something else for at least fifteen minutes. If you still feel hungry after fifteen minutes, have a large glass of water. If your hunger has still not subsided, have more vegetables, salad or some fresh fruit.

Pull up a chair

Where you eat will also impact your weight. Studies show that the best place to eat is sitting down at the table while doing nothing else. Why? You want to focus on the food and its flavor. When you eat while working on the computer, reading the newspaper, watching the TV or playing with your phone, your fullness may not register as quickly. That can lead to overeating and make it harder to lose weight. Did you ever eat something and think to yourself...hmm...now where did it go and I want more?

Distractions from eating can lead to overeating and make it harder to lose weight. At your next meal take the time to sit down at the table and enjoy what you are eating. Focus on practicing the five steps to eating slowly (above) and truly experience how eating slower will allow you to enjoy the pleasure of tasting the food and, overall, help you eat less.

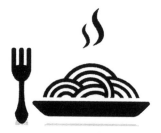

Swap your plate

Do you eat from a large dinner plate? Do you put cereal in a large soup bowl or a small bowl? Using smaller plates and bowls, and even small spoons and forks (yes, the teaspoon and salad fork!) has been shown to help people eat less. So make smart swaps for smaller utensils and eat less without even realizing it!

Are you hungry?

Before you reach for a snack or sit down for a meal, do you ask yourself how hungry you are? If you don't, try starting now. Learning to eat when you are at the right level of hunger can help you avoid emotional or mindless eating. Emotional hunger is a need to eat to fill an emotional void, which may be caused by boredom, loneliness or stress. True hunger is when your blood glucose (or blood sugar) is decreasing and your body needs food for energy to bring it back up.

One way to think about your hunger level is to use a **Hunger Chart**. I've seen the Hunger Chart help teens become more aware of what they eat and when they eat it—to ultimately help them eat less. It will help you decide whether you're truly hungry, desiring food for emotional reasons, or just because you know it's available in your fridge. Based on a scale of 1 to 10 (with 1 being very hungry and 10 being full to the point of nausea), you can tell whether it is sensible for you to eat now or wait. As a general rule, eat when you're at 3 or 4 and stop eating when you're at 6 or 7.

Check out the following Hunger Chart.

Hunger Chart

1. *Faint with hunger/shaking*
2. *Feeling starving*
3. *Reasonably hungry*
4. *Slightly hungry*
5. *Not hungry/content*
6. *Pleasantly content*
7. *Full*
8. *Very full*
9. *Bloated/gassy from excess food*
10. *Nauseous from excessive eating*

What can you do if you are an emotional eater?
Are you an emotional eater? You may not be sure whether you eat for emotional reasons. Keeping a daily food log in a notebook or on your phone is a good way to find out. Here's what to write down each day:

*What you ate and the approximate time
*How much you ate
*"Feelings" column (to write down your emotions)

Sample Food Log

Meal	Time	Food	Amount	How did you feel?
Breakfast				
Lunch				
Snack				
Dinner				

Why does emotional eating matter?

You probably know that food may make you feel better while you're eating it, when sad, stressed or lonely. But not long after, you see that your pre-food feelings are still there *and* you've eaten **a lot** of calories you don't need. Mentally, as well as physically, you may feel worse. If you realize you aren't always hungry when you eat, it may be time to either see a counselor for help or address it on your own (if you think you can). Whenever you feel the urge to eat and you aren't at Level 3 on the Hunger Chart, plan to get out of the kitchen and do something else. Exercise is a terrific way to reduce stress.

Give one or more of these a try to help avoid emotional eating:

*Go for a walk or take an exercise class at your local gym.
*Put on some music and dance.
*Get a hobby: You may find that you love to paint, knit, or write.
*Keep a daily journal to help lift your spirits.
*If you have a dog, take him or her for a walk.
*Pick up a book, sit in a comfortable chair and sip a cup of herb tea to help calm anger and/or frustration.
*Call a friend or family member for emotional support.

It takes practice, but you can learn to eat **only** when you are physically hungry. Jot down ideas for non-food activities you enjoy in your food log. Check there first when you're looking for something to help you deal with feeling sad, angry, stressed, lonely or bored.

Avoid Food Portion Distortion

Do you know what a portion is? It's a good idea to start getting familiar with standard food portions from each food group. Then you'll know how much to serve yourself or eat from your plate—whether preparing your own meal, choosing a snack, having dinner in a restaurant or someone else's home. You may have been to many restaurants that serve you enough food to feed three or four people. And quite often when you read the serving size on a single-serve snack bag, though it says it is one serving, the serving is two or more portions! Knowing portion sizes will help you recognize when this happens.

A proper portion of food may seem like a small difference—say, 100 fewer calories. But if you cut just 100 calories per day, you can lose ten pounds in a year. So do yourself a favor and start getting to know portion sizes: **Make sure to have measuring cups and spoons in your kitchen drawer at home.** Use them when preparing a meal or snack.

Test yourself tomorrow morning: Do you really know what a serving of your favorite cereal looks like? Read the cereal box label for the serving size and number of calories. Pour it into a bowl and then measure back into the measuring cup (before you add the milk!). One cup or less will do just fine! Those small food scales sold in department or housewares stores can come in handy for measuring ounces of meat, fish, chicken and cheese. Once you know what a standard portion looks like you won't need to continue measuring. Portion control is key!

Measuring cups and spoons are also helpful for both measuring ingredients when you are cooking as well as to keep you on track with standard portions. You don't have to measure everything you eat **forever**. But the more you measure now, the more confident you'll be in evaluating your plate. If you are still hungry when you finish your meal go back for more vegetables or salad. Vegetables, in addition to being powerhouses of vitamins and minerals, are low in calories, (unless they are loaded with oil or butter), high in fiber and quite filling.

Standard Portions of Food vs. Serving Size on the Package

Just an FYI: You should know that the standard portion and what is printed on the Nutrition Fact label is not always the same. Quite often the serving size in the package can be double or more the standard portion size. Remember those lunch-packs of Oreos that contained six cookies when the portion size is **only two**? Who ate just two!! If you familiarize yourself with standard portions you'll be more likely to stay on track with how much you are eating.

So, what should you be measuring? An excellent (and free!) app for portion sizes and nutrition information is Calorie King. **Start with these standard portions**:

Protein sources

Meat, fish chicken: 3 ounces cooked (This is about the size of a deck of cards.)
Tofu: 8 ounces
Beans: 1 cup
Nut butter: 2 tablespoon
Cheese: 1 1/2 ounces cheese
Cottage cheese: 1/2 cup (4 ounces)
Egg: 2 eggs or 4 egg whites
Hummus: 4 tablespoons

Dairy

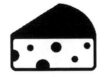

Milk, calcium-fortified soy or almond milk: 1 cup
Yogurt: 1 cup
Cheese: 1.5 ounces

Non-starchy Vegetables

Vegetables (such as broccoli, Brussels sprouts, cauliflower, eggplant and zucchini): 1 cup raw or 1/2 cup, cooked
Lettuce or other salad greens: 1 cup

Starchy Vegetables

Beans: 1/2 cup
Corn: 1 ear or 1/2 cup
Peas: 1/2 cup
Potato, white: 1 small
Potato, sweet: 1/2 cup
Butternut and acorn squash: 1/2 cup

Fruit

Fresh or frozen fruit: 1/2 cup or 1 small fruit
Dried fruit: approx. 1/4 cup (depends on fruit size) raisins: 2 tbsp
Juice (100% juice): 1/2 cup or 4 ounces

Grains

Cereal: 1/2 to 1 cup
Cooked pasta/rice: 1/3 cup Usual portion=1 to 2 cups (be aware–
this equals 3 to 6 servings)
Bread: 1 slice (1 ounce)
Bagel: 1 bagel equals about 4 to 8 servings of bread
Mini-bagel: = 2 slices bread
Large roll: = 4 slices bread

Fats

Oil: 1 teaspoon
Butter: 1 teaspoon
Olives: 5
Avocado: 1/4 of an avocado

Step 3. Stay on Track with Self-Monitoring

Self-monitoring simply means keeping track of your progress towards a healthy lifestyle. Researchers have found that people who use self-monitoring tools **lose more weight** and are more likely to keep it off than those who don't use them. I recommend two of these tools for teens losing weight:

1. Keeping a daily food and exercise log
2. Weighing yourself once a week

You can use one or both of these strategies to help you stay focused, self-aware and, ultimately, reach your weight loss goal. There's an added benefit: Whether you're seeing the good food choices you've made listed on paper (or your phone) or seeing the number on the scale drop by the month, you'll be inspired to keep moving toward a healthier lifestyle.

1. Keeping a Daily Food and Exercise Log

Many studies have shown that people lose **more** weight when they keep a daily food and exercise log or journal. Writing down what you eat throughout the day will help you see when you are doing well and where you could make improvements in your food choices. You may notice you want to make healthy changes by changing your snack foods or portion sizes, for example. If you also record the time when you eat, you may notice that skipping a meal or waiting too long to eat may cause you to get too hungry and overeat. Writing down when you exercise and how long you're active will also help you as you keep track of your weight loss progress.

Yep, There's an App For That! Use Apps for daily food and exercise logs.

Don't like to write? Check out some apps and websites to keep your daily log. These can make the job quicker and easier. Have you tried searching for apps to track your eating and exercise? For starters, LoseIt and MyFitnessPal are popular, free, and available for iPhones and iPads. You can record what you eat as well as your exercise routine and these apps will keep track. You can also have LoseIt text you when you forget to log in you meals and snacks. Please check **Part 3. Tools of the Trade** for a list of apps and websites to help you reach your weight and health goals.

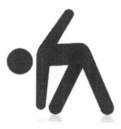

Please see the following **food and exercise log**. If you want to keep a daily food log in a notebook, you can use a format such as this.

Daily Food and Activity Log
Instructions: Please include the time you ate, the foods and beverages you had and the amount eaten. Also include the type of exercise you did and the amount of time you spent performing this activity.

	M	T	W	T	F	S	S
Breakfast							
Lunch							
Snack							
Dinner							
Exercise							

To Weigh or Not Weigh?

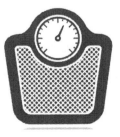

The most important thing to remember about this question is: *The answer is up to you!* Whatever you find to be helpful or motivating. Here's how to decide whether to step on the scale **once a week**: **If knowing your weight makes you feel overwhelmed or discouraged,** hold off from weighing for now. Start to make some healthy changes in the foods you eat and try to exercise for one hour each day.

As you feel your clothes getting looser, you may be ready to get on the scale and see what you weigh. Being aware of your weight and seeing the results of your hard work can motivate you. And noticing how your body feels better may increase your motivation to fuel your body well. Then it may be easier to make healthy food choices. You will be more likely to choose raw vegetables and hummus or fresh fruit for a snack instead of a chocolate glazed donut or a piece of cake! Always remember: Eat well to feel well!

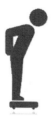

When should I weigh?

If you want to keep track of your weight, weigh yourself once per week. Be consistent–if you weigh yourself on Thursday morning, try to always weigh yourself on Thursday morning. Don't get obsessed with the number you see; that can set you up for eating problems down the road. Instead use the number on the scale as a way to measure your progress. Losing weight is for your health. It's not a contest! Many times you may think you gained back at least five pounds, especially after vacation or a holiday. You may not want to get on the scale. Your clothes feel tight. Then you get on the scale and see that it is only an extra one or two pounds—or you stayed at the same weight! Everyone's weight fluctuates. Knowing your weight means you're more likely to prevent weight regain. When you notice you've gone up a few pounds, it's much easier to make small changes to your food and activity levels to drop the extra weight. The key is to use the scale as a tool to stay aware and keep moving toward your goal.

How much weight is healthy to lose? Because you are a teen, you may still be growing. Therefore you don't want to lose weight quickly as it can jeopardize your potential growth in height. Be aware that we all lose weight at different rates depending upon many factors, which may include your body size (or frame) amount of extra weight, food intake, genetics plus intensity and frequency of exercise. So try to limit your weight loss to one pound per week. That may not sound like a lot, but over the course of one year, depending on your weight loss goals, one pound per week can add up to 52 pounds! Thus if you want to lose twenty pounds, give yourself at least five months or twenty weeks to realize your weight loss goal. If you lose weight slower, it is more likely to be sustainable. When you lose weight slowly, you give yourself more time to learn new eating behaviors **and** then they are more likely to last!

Step 4. Exercise: Move It if You Want to Lose It!

Getting Exercise Every Day
Research shows that almost everyone who keeps weight off has one thing in common: **They exercise**. Not only can exercise help you lose weight and maintain your weight loss, but you will reap the rewards of so many other benefits including:

improved energy levels
increased ability to handle stress
improved mood
reduced risk of many chronic diseases
enhanced self-esteem
more positive outlook on life in general

So try to make a habit of getting at least one hour of exercise each day. The easiest way to start? Find something you like to do. Make exercise a **fun** part of your day! Read on for some ideas.

How to Get Your Hour of Exercise

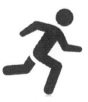

Start walking: Exercise doesn't have to mean running fast or feeling uncomfortable. The easiest way to exercise is to walk. For starters, get a pedometer and set it to zero each morning when you get out of bed. The pedometer counts every step you take. Aim for 10,000 steps per day. (That equals five miles!) Do you have a friend who will join you for regular walks? Make a plan to meet at a designated time several times per week.

Do you have a dog? Then take your pet for a fast-paced walk. If not, you can still walk or run around your neighborhood solo. Listening to an iPod can help pass the time. If you like to walk, this simple mode of fitness will help you burn calories and lose weight.

Pop in an exercise DVD*:* Is walking too slow? Don't enjoy the gym or exercise classes? There are still plenty of other ways to get your exercise fix! One easy strategy is to pick up a few exercise DVDs and work out at home. Your local library or video store will usually have a nice supply of exercise videos for you to try out before you make a purchase. Check out a few and see what you like. You can also find some terrific DVDs on the internet. Two great websites to purchase exercise videos are www.collagevideo.com and www.overstock.com.

Mix it up: If you like to dance, get moving by signing up for a dance class like jazz, tap, or even high-energy Zumba (find classes near you at www.zumba.com). Or ride your bike. Tennis, rollerblading and swimming are also fun ways to get moving. The choices are endless. My favorite exercise is kickboxing. Walking my dog each morning for at least thirty minutes is another way I get in more exercise. And if I have extra time in the afternoon, I try to get in another two-mile walk. If you find that you love many different types of exercise like me, do a variety! It sure beats boredom. Another big plus is that a varied exercise routine works all of your muscle groups.

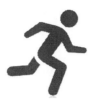

Plan your week: The key to consistent exercise? Plan a weekly schedule and stick with it. **Try to get in some activity every day, for a total of at least four hours per week.** And you don't have to do one hour all at once. You can exercise in 15 minute increments 4 times a day if that works better for you. If you plan workouts for four days, take a more relaxed approach to activity on the other three days. Perhaps you'll take your dog for an extended walk, ride your bike, or put on some music and dance in your bedroom. Whatever you do—just enjoy it!

Benefits of Regular Exercise

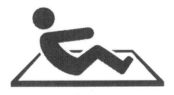

Why do so many health experts recommend an hour of exercise each day? Just check out the benefits:

> **Exercise improves every part of the body, including the mind.** Exercising produces endorphins, which are chemicals that can help you feel happy and relaxed. It may also help those with mild depression and poor self-esteem. Exercise may also help you sleep better. In addition, achieving exercise goals, such as walking two miles every day, can give you a real sense of accomplishment.

Exercising can help you look better. Exercise decreases body fat, builds muscle mass and makes your body more toned.

Exercise helps people lose weight and lowers the risk of some diseases. Exercising to maintain a healthy weight lowers your risk of developing certain diseases including type 2 diabetes and high blood pressure. These diseases used to be seen primarily in adults, but are now becoming more common in teens.

Exercise can help a person age well. This may not seem important now, but your body will thank you later. Women are especially prone (but males can develop it as well) to a condition called osteoporosis (thinning of the bones) as they get older. Your bones reach their peak between the ages of 25 and 30. During the teen years is the time to build strong bones. Studies have found that weight-bearing exercise, such as jumping, running, walking and lifting weights can help teens keep their bones strong.

A well-rounded exercise program should include the following: 1) aerobic exercise, 2) strength training and 3) flexibility training. Let's take a look at each type of exercise and see how you can easily make them part of your exercise routine.

Aerobic Exercise

Like other muscles, your heart enjoys a good workout. Give it one in the form of aerobic exercise. Aerobic exercise, also referred to as cardio exercise, is any type of exercise that gets the heart pumping and quickens your breathing. When you give your heart this kind of workout on a regular basis, it will get stronger and more efficient in delivering oxygen to all parts of your body. If you play team sports, you're probably meeting the recommendation for 60 minutes or more of moderate to vigorous activity on practice days. Some team sports that give you a great cardio workout are lacrosse, basketball, soccer, hockey and rowing.

To start an aerobic exercise program, just put on your sneakers and start walking. It's fun—and free. You can walk in your neighborhood or at the school track. If walking is not your thing, grab your bike and start riding, jump rope, or try a fitness app such as Nike Training Club. Or try them all!

Here are some other ways to get cardio exercise on your own or with friends: biking, running, swimming, dancing, tennis, cross-country skiing, hiking, and power walking.

Cardio exercise provides numerous health benefits. Many aerobic exercises are also "weight-bearing"—the kind where you stand on your feet to exercise. Weight-bearing cardio exercises include walking, aerobics, dancing, tennis, climbing stairs, and running. These types of exercise stimulates the cells that make new bone and boost bone strength. Aerobic exercise may also help reduce your risk of developing diabetes, heart disease and some types of cancer. In fact, the aerobic exercise that you can do on your own such as running, power walking, etc., will be easier to continue when you leave high school and go on to college or a job, so you can stay fit for life.

Last but not least, **aerobic exercise is your key to maintaining a normal weight**. It reduces your belly fat and even lessens stress. Studies show that high levels of hormones, such as cortisol, which your body releases when it feels stress may be the cause of belly fat. And what's one of the best stress relievers? Exercise!

2) Strength Training

The heart isn't the only muscle to benefit from regular exercise. When you strengthen all of your body's muscles by exercising, it allows you to stay active longer without getting tired. Strong muscles also support your joints and help to prevent injuries in daily life. **And here's the key for weight loss:** All of your body tissues burn calories for energy, even when you're not moving. But your muscles burn more calories than fat does, so building more muscle mass with strength training helps with weight control. Exercise is a "win-win" situation!

Different types of exercise strengthens different muscle groups. Try some of these to help develop your muscles:

> **For building arm muscles:** try push-ups and planks. You can also purchase three- or five-pound weights and do arm exercises at home.

For strong legs: try fast walking, running, biking and skating. Squats, lunges, and leg raises also work the legs.

For well-developed abs (think six-pack!): crunches, yoga, or Pilates are ideal.

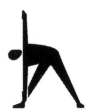

3) Flexibility Training

Quite often people don't take the time to stretch their muscles **after** their workout. But you should enjoy a good stretch. To bend over, pick up your dog, clean up your room or just to get out of bed, you need flexibility. If you take just a few minutes to stretch after your workout, you can greatly increase your mobility and reduce the risk of chronic injuries as you get older.

Some people are naturally more flexible. Flexibility is primarily related to genetics, gender, age and level of physical activity. We tend to lose flexibility as we grow older, usually due to inactivity rather than the aging process itself. The less active we are, the less flexible we tend to be. As with aerobic endurance and strength training, flexibility will improve the more often you stretch.

How can I work stretching into my workout?
Flexibility training includes stretching exercises. Yoga is one popular way—you can probably find a class offered nearby. Or download a yoga app onto your phone. Not only can yoga make you more flexible, it's also a great way to manage stress levels.

Ideally, spend at least 30 minutes, three times per week, on flexibility training. But even five minutes of stretching at the end of **every** exercise session is better than nothing. To start, include at least a few minutes of stretching **after** your aerobic or resistance training. You'll feel more relaxed and rejuvenated.

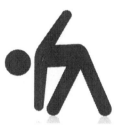

Feel like you just don't have time to stretch? Here are some tips for fitting stretching into an overstuffed schedule:

1. Try simple stretches before getting out of bed in the morning. Sit back on your legs and stretch your arms forward on the bed.

2. Try a few full-body stretches when you wake up: stand up straight, tighten your abdominal muscles and reach your arms above your head. This can help kick start your morning.

3. Take a stretching class such as yoga or tai chi. Scheduling a class will help you stick with a regular program. You can also get yoga or tai chi DVDs and apps to do at home. Go to www. yogadownload.com for free 20-minute classes.

10 Tips to Make Exercise Part of Your Daily Routine

1. Turn your pedometer on each morning and aim for 10,000 steps per day. It is quite motivating to chart your progress throughout the day.

2. Put aside one hour each day and MOVE! Turn on the music and dance.

3. Walk to and/or home from school.

4. Park your car farther away in the parking lot.

5. Walk your dog at least 30 minutes each day.

6. Sign up for an exercise class at your local YMCA.

7. Take out some exercise DVDs from the library. Find one you like, buy it and use it!

8. Use the Wii for exercise.

9. Take a walk at your local park, beach or mall.

10. Sign up for a local community walk/run and start to train. For a training plan, check out the Couch to 5K walking and jogging program at www.c25k.com.

Recommended Exercise Apps

Nike Training Club (free for iPhone)

Recommended DVDs

Leslie Sansone Walking DVDs (www.lesliesansone.com) These videos are great–you can easily walk a mile or more in your bedroom!)

Zumba class (www.zumba.com)

Step 5. Don't Drink Your Calories: Be Beverage Savvy!

Where's the water?

Did you know that water makes up more than two-thirds–about 66%– of your body weight? The water in your body supplies fluid for saliva and tears, keeps your temperature normal, flushes waste products from your liver and kidneys and helps prevent constipation. Clearly, water is essential for good health and for feeling good.

Many people make the mistake of getting the fluids we need during the day from sodas, flavored milk, fancy coffee beverages, and juices. These drinks are high in calories from sugar, so they can increase your caloric intake which can add on pounds (or make it harder to lose weight).

Check out the following beverage chart:

Beverage	Serving Size	Calories	Amount of sugar
Juice	1 cup (8 ounces)	120	8 teaspoons
Soda	1 can (12 ounces)	150	10 teaspoons
Frappuccino	Tall (12 ounces)	180	9 teaspoons
Chocolate milk	1 cup (8 ounces)	150	6 teaspoons
Water	**1 cup (8 ounces)**	**0**	**0 teaspoons**

Why is water the best beverage choice?

Water is the best thing you can drink—hands down. It is nearly always free from a nearby faucet. Most importantly, it's the best thirst-quencher, and calorie free.

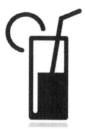

What if you don't like to drink water?

Here's a few ways to make sure drinking water doesn't feel like a chore:

1. Seltzer water is another healthy drink that has the fizzy feel of soda without any calories. Instead of diet soda, try seltzer and a squeeze of lemon or lime with your meal.
2. Have herbal teas brewed hot, or use them to make homemade iced tea.
3. If you like a little sweetness in your drink, try 1 teaspoon or 1 packet sugar (just 16 calories) or stevia (a calorie-free, herbal sweetener that is safe to use). Sweeten iced tea or fresh lemonade (made with fresh lemon and ice water) using stevia for a calorie-free drink.
4. Crystal Lite Pure is a new beverage sweetened with stevia, has 15 calories per 8 ounce serving and doesn't contain artificial colors or flavors.

Why isn't diet soda recommended as a beverage? There is some evidence that drinking diet sodas may cause weight gain by increasing your taste for additional sweets. Thus if you do like to drink diet soda, try to limit it to 1 serving or can per day.

For good health try to limit added sugar (from all sources of foods and beverages) to a maximum of six teaspoons per day.

Thirst vs. Hunger

Sometimes drinking a glass of water quells your hunger. It's easy to mix up feelings of hunger and thirst, so have a drink before grabbing a snack. It can help you eat less food. Pay special attention to your thirst if you think you're hungry, but it's only been two hours (or less) since your last meal. Sometimes we eat, when we're not truly hungry, simply because we're bored.

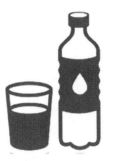

What happens if you don't drink enough?

You lose water every day through bodily functions (sweating, urinating). These water losses need to be replenished so you don't get dehydrated, which can slow you down. Here's what can happen if you don't drink enough water every day:

-You can get problems such as palpitations (irregular heart beat) or feel very tired.
-You may notice that you often get a headache later in the day.
-Digested food stays in your intestine—leading to gas, constipation and bloating. On the other hand, drinking water pushes digested food through your intestine.

How do I know if I'm well hydrated?

An easy way is to look at your urine. If it is dark yellow, you may be dehydrated. But if it's a pale straw color or almost colorless, you are getting enough water.

How much water do you need per day?

Research has not shown us exactly how much water each person should drink every day. But in general, 8 to 9 cups of fluid should be enough. (When I say "fluid," that means water and other drinks like seltzer and tea, and even soups.) If you sweat a lot because you're active or live in a warm climate, you probably need even more than 8-9 cups. So how can you stay on track? Here are two strategies that have worked for teens I know:

Try to drink two cups of fluid with each meal.

Try to drink at least 1 cup of fluid with each snack.

Having a fluid routine like this will help you stay on track, just like your meal routine.

Besides drinking water, where does water in our diets come from?

Water is in many foods, including soups, milk, tea, coffee, and juices. Many fruits and vegetables also contain a fair amount of water. If you have a cup of soup or milk with your meal, count it as 1 cup of water. Try not to drink juice since it's high in sugar and calories. One orange is equal to ½ cup juice, but juice fills you up the same as water. Plus, juice has no fiber—you'll be fuller if you eat the piece of fruit instead.

The Lowdown on Alcohol and Your Weight

The legal U.S. drinking age is 21, but I know that some teens drink. I'm not here to preach to you. My goal is to 1) help keep you healthy and 2) help you lose weight. With those goals in mind, I want you to remember a few things:

Staying healthy: Alcohol can damage your liver and make you sick.

Losing weight: Alcohol has 7 calories per gram. These "empty calories" can add up quickly and impact your weight loss. Did you know drinking alcohol can lower your blood sugar? Low blood sugar can make you hungry, leading to excess snacking and, ultimately, weight gain.

Ten Tips to Increase Your Fluid Intake

1. Squeeze fresh lemon or lime into your water to give it a little zing.
2. Add sliced fruit to a pitcher of water for a hint of sweetness.
3. Snack on fruits and veggies high in water like watermelon, tomatoes, cucumbers and celery.
4. Begin each meal or snack with a glass of water. It adds up.
5. Always carry a water bottle with you. You'll drink more.
6. Start the day off right with a glass of water as soon as you wake up.
7. To relax after dinner, have a cup of herbal tea.
8. Have nonfat milk or soymilk on your cereal or in your smoothie.
9. Get in the habit of having a broth-based soup to start your dinner.
10. Drink iced herbal tea if it will help you drink more.

Step 6. Cut Down on the Sugar (aka Get Rid of The Junk)

Now you're ready to learn how to eat healthy and lose weight. So where should you begin? Start by *slowly* losing the junk food. That's foods like soda, candy, chips, doughnuts, sugary cakes and cookies. They taste good, but give you lots of "empty" calories— calories without the nutrients you need. They're also high in sugar or white flour (or many times, both), which makes them low in fiber and quick to digest.

So what happens when you eat junk food? Your blood sugar jumps up and then goes down quickly. While it's on its way down, your brain is already starting to tell your stomach it's time to eat. Soon you'll feel hungry—you may have felt this happen—and you start to crave *more* sugar. It's easy to see why eating lots of sugary foods won't help you meet your weight goals.

When you want to have something sweet, grab a piece of fruit. Whether it's a juicy orange, a crunchy apple, or tart, fresh raspberries, you'll be getting vitamins, minerals, and fiber, too. The fiber will help you feel full and stay full for at least one hour. If you combine the fruit with a protein such as 10 nuts or 1 cheese stick, you may find yourself staying full for three hours or more! Since it does have some sugar, stick to three or four servings of fruit per day. (One serving is about a half cup of cut fruit or a small piece of whole fruit, like a banana or apple.) If you want to spice up your fruit snack, try dipping sliced fruit in nonfat vanilla or lemon yogurt or adding a sprinkle of cinnamon to chopped apples.

How does too much sugar impact my weight and health?

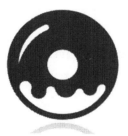

The average teen consumes 28 teaspoons of added sugar per day. This translates to 476 calories or about 25% of your daily calorie needs! That much sugar makes it hard to lose weight, and eating a high-sugar diet may increase your risk for diabetes in the future. It also increases your risk for developing heart disease, high blood pressure, and some types of cancer.

Have you ever noticed that sugar can also make you feel tired?

Picture this: You have a lot of studying to do for your exam tomorrow. After a healthy lunch at school, you have a can of Coke with a candy bar around 4 p.m. Then you sit down in your comfortable chair, get your laptop out, and open up your notes. Within thirty minutes, it's hard to keep your eyes open. The sugary soda and candy gave you quick energy, but your blood sugar dropped—**fast** and your energy level tanked.

To keep your energy up, you want to mix complex carbohydrates (like whole grain crackers, a granola bar, such as Kashi TLC or a fruit and protein (like hummus, peanut butter, or low-fat cheese). Try a combo of these before your next study session and see how you feel.

Interesting Fact: Drinking one 12-ounce soda per day over the course of one year adds up to 50 pounds of sugar. Yikes!

How do I start cutting down on sugar?

You might be surprised by just how much sugar you can cut out with two simple swaps. Teens often use these strategies to start eating less sugar:

1. **Swap the candy for fresh fruit.** Instead of Oreos for dessert, go for a fresh orange or a small dish of fresh pineapple. Or put a cup of frozen fruit in the blender and make sorbet!
2. **Drink water in place of the sugary drinks**. Instead of soda or juice at lunch, bring a stainless-steel water bottle filled with cold water from home.

You might not think you eat or drink a lot of sugar. But sugar can sneak in when you're not paying attention. To find out, keep a food record for three days. Look at the labels of the foods and beverages you consume. Jot down the number of grams of added sugar in each food or drink you have. At the end of the day, review how many sugary drinks, teaspoons or packets of sugar you added to your food and beverages (one teaspoon or packet of sugar = 4 grams), sweetened cereals, cookies, sweetened yogurts, and granola bars you consumed. Tally up the sugar grams, and divide by four—this is the number of teaspoons of sugar you had that day.

Just an FYI: Try to avoid products that contain any form of sugar within the first three ingredients on the packages' ingredient label. Sugar may be listed as sweetener, syrup or have the suffix "ose."

Avoid fruit juice. Juices don't contain any fiber. Plus they are high in sugar and calories.

For good health try to limit added sugar to a maximum of six teaspoons per day.

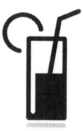

Stevia: A Healthy Non-Caloric Sweetener

A healthy alternative to sugar is stevia. Stevia is a sweetener made from a plant and has no harmful side effects. One packet of stevia is as sweet as two teaspoons of sugar. But unlike sugar, which has 16 calories per teaspoon, stevia has 0 calories. Add just a small amount and adjust as needed. Stevia is found in the grocery store in the sugar aisle. Try adding a small amount to plain oatmeal, yogurt and iced tea for a little extra sweetness instead of buying foods with added sugar. You can also make your own fresh lemonade with water, a squeeze of fresh lemon and a half teaspoon of stevia or one teaspoon of sugar.

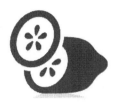

Decrease Your Sweet Tooth with These Sugar Swaps

Instead of this:	Try this:
Soda	Water or seltzer, For more flavor add stevia and/or lemon
Sugary cereals	Cheerios or Shredded Wheat. If you want sweetness add 1 tsp. sugar or stevia or some fresh fruit. Healthy cereals have 6 grams of sugar or less and at least 3 grams of fiber.
Juices or bottled lemonade or tea	Water, seltzer or plain iced tea. Make fresh lemonade with water, fresh lemon and 1 tsp. sugar or stevia.
Sugary jams, jellies and syrup	Fresh cup-up bananas or berries on peanut butter sandwiches, waffles and pancakes

Sweetened yogurt	Add your own fresh fruit to plain yogurt. if you want more sweetness, add 1 tsp. sugar or stevia. A typical 8 ounce yogurt has 4 teaspoons sugar!
Candy bar	Granola bar such as Kashi, Lara or Kind. Or make your own trail mix: Put 2 Tbsp. each nuts and whole grain cereal and 1 Tbsp. dried fruit in a baggie. Make a bunch and grab one each morning as you run out the door.
Ice cream or frozen yogurt	Frozen fruit. Slice a ripe banana or take a small bunch of grapes or berries, put in a baggie and freeze. Pineapple is also delicious frozen.
Cookies	Grab a fresh apple or orange.
Cake or pie	Fresh fruit salad or plain yogurt and fresh fruit. YUM!

Step 7. Fill Up on Fiber

Many teens ask me which foods will help them feel full without going over their calorie needs. My advice: **Fill your plate with fiber.** You can only get fiber (also known as "dietary fiber") from plant foods. It's not naturally found in meat or dairy. Plant foods include fruits and vegetables, whole grains, including breads and cereals, beans, nuts, and seeds.

First, a few types of fiber to understand: All dietary fiber found in plant foods is either **soluble** or **insoluble**. These types of fiber differ in how they react with water. Soluble fiber dissolves in water to form a gel-like substance. It helps stabilize blood sugar and lower cholesterol. Soluble fiber includes beans, oats, apples and bananas. Insoluble fiber attracts water and is known for promoting regularity in the intestinal tract. Insoluble fiber is found in whole wheat, bran, nuts, seeds and the peel of some fruits and vegetables. If you eat a variety of plant foods, you'll get a mix of soluble and insoluble fibers, which are both good for your health. "Functional fibers," such as inulin, come from plant sources or may be commercially synthesized, such as polydextrose. Food companies add functional fibers to packaged foods, such as yogurt and granola bars. All fiber is healthy for you, but research shows that fiber from whole foods (rather than fiber added to processed foods) helps you lose the most weight. This finding is likely because high-fiber whole foods—such as fruits, vegetables, and beans—are also low in calories. Fiber alone won't melt off the pounds. You still need to eat a healthy, calorie-controlled meal plan and get regular physical activity. But it's easier to control or maintain your weight when you eat plenty of fiber.

What else can fiber do for my health? Fiber does more than just manage your weight. Having a diet rich in fiber will:

-Help promote regular bowel movements, thus avoiding constipation.

-Decrease your risk of developing diabetes, diverticulosis, constipation, irritable bowel syndrome and colon cancer.

-Slow down the digestion of sugar and keep blood sugar more stable.

-Reduce your risk for heart disease. Why? Fiber that you eat ends up in your intestine, where it binds to cholesterol (a type of fat) and then is eliminated, so you absorb less cholesterol into your bloodstream.

Read on to find out how to get fiber from the foods you eat.

How much fiber should I eat daily?

Aim for somewhere in **between 25 and 35 grams** of dietary fiber per day. You can make it easy to reach this goal by eating about seven grams of fiber at each meal and three grams of fiber at each snack. Remember the MyPlate method (www.myplate.gov) from Step 1? If you're filling half your plate with fruits and vegetables —and another quarter of your plate with whole grains—at breakfast, lunch, and dinner, getting enough fiber will come naturally.

If you're eating a packaged food, check the Nutrition Facts label for the number of fiber grams per serving. For example, if you have two servings of fruit (8 grams) and 3 servings vegetables (9 grams of fiber), one serving of beans (8 grams), and three servings of whole grain (9 grams) per day, you will be consuming about 34 grams of dietary fiber. Read the following list to get a better idea of the amount of fiber in common foods.

Which foods have fiber? Examples of foods that have fiber include:

Grains, breads, and cereals

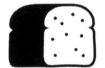

Brown rice, 1/2 cup cooked	2.0 grams
Quinoa, 1/3 cup cooked	3.0 grams
Whole wheat pasta (1/2 cup cooked)	3.0 grams
1 whole-wheat English muffin	4.4 grams
1 slice whole grain bread	2.0 grams
Whole-grain cereal, cold:	
1/2 cup of All-Bran	9.6 grams
3/4 cup of Total	2.4 grams
1 cup Cheerios	3.0 grams
1 packet of whole-grain cereal, hot:	
(oatmeal, Wheatena)	3.0 grams

Fruits

1 medium apple, with skin	3.3 grams
1 medium pear, with skin	4.3 grams
1 cup of raspberries	8.0 grams
1 banana	3.1 grams
1 cup strawberries	2.9 grams
1 orange, medium	3.1 grams
1 cup blueberries	3.5 grams
1 cup pineapple	2.2 grams

Vegetables (Starchy and Non-Starchy)

1/2 cup of chickpeas	8.0 grams
1/2 cup of kidney beans	8.2 grams
1/2 cup of black beans	7.5 grams
1/2 cup of winter squash	2.9 grams
1 medium sweet potato with skin	4.8 grams
1/2 cup of green peas	4.4 grams
1 medium potato with skin	3.8 grams
1 cup of cauliflower	2.5 grams
1/2 cup of spinach	3.5 grams
1/2 cup of turnip greens	2.5 grams

Source: Adapted from U.S. Department of Agriculture and U.S. Department of Health and Human Services, *Dietary Guidelines for Americans*, 2005

How do I add fiber to my diet?
The key is to add fiber <u>slowly</u>. This gives your body time to adapt so you avoid gas and bloating. Another tip to steer clear of gas or constipation: Drink more water as you up the fiber. Fiber **needs** fluid to help it move through your intestinal tract. Always aim for

at least eight cups of fluid per day. To see how much fiber you are now consuming keep a food record and add up the amount of fiber you are **now** eating in one day. Then add five grams of fiber—which is equivalent to one fruit or 2 slices of whole grain bread—into your daily meal routine each day for one week. At the second week add in **another** five grams of fiber per day and so on, until you reach a minimum of twenty-five grams of fiber per day.

The **key** to getting more fiber into your diet is to emphasize more plant-based foods in their natural form:

Choose whole grain cereals and breads instead of refined white breads and cereals. Good choices for whole grain cereals that are also low in sugar are Plain or Multigrain Cheerios, Kashi Heart to Heart and Barbara's Cinnamon Puffins. Whole grains are rich in fiber, whereas the fiber is removed from white bread, semolina pasta, white rice and many cereals during processing.

Check the labels on food products. When you look at the ingredient list, the first word should be "whole" (for example, "whole wheat" or "whole grain oats."). Also check the Nutrition Facts label for the number of grams under "Dietary Fiber." *At least* two grams per serving in a grain-based food, like breads or crackers, is a good sign. Check out the following label:

Ingredients:

Whole Grain Oats Modified Corn
Starch, Corn Starch, Sugar, Salt,
Tocopherols, Trisodium Phosphate,
Calcium Carbonate, Natural Colour.
Contains Wheat Ingredients.

Go for raw or cooked veggies, which are full of fiber and nutrients but low in calories. Make sure you fill up on vegetables at lunch and dinner. At least one half of your plate should be vegetables. Check out www.myplate.gov for more info on choosing a healthy plate.

Choose whole fruit (fresh, frozen or dried) instead of canned fruits and juices. Fresh, frozen and dried fruits contain more fiber than canned fruit.

Limit dried fruit to one serving per day. Dried fruit also contains fiber, but the fluid has been taken out so you can eat a lot more before you feel full. So you must watch the amount you eat carefully: One ounce dried (about 1/4 cup) equals one fruit serving.

Avoid fruit juice. Juices don't contain any fiber. They are high in sugar and calories and fill you the same as water!

The bottom line Here's an analogy I like to share with teens: One small orange or apple (about 60 calories) usually has fewer calories than one cookie (75 to 100 calories). And a serving of fresh fruit will fill you up. You know one cookie won't. That's because it has no fiber.

The same goes for juice: A ½-cup of juice is also equivalent to a small orange (both have 60 calories). But drinking the juice is like drinking a glass of water—it won't fill you for long plus it contains calories and sugar. Go for the fresh fruit to get fuller, stay satisfied and manage your weight.

Meet Your Fiber Quota: 10 Tips to Eat More Fiber

Not sure where to begin? Start with one of these tips to get more fiber:

1. Choose whole grains instead of refined (white) grains. Enjoy whole grain breads, pastas, brown rice, quinoa, whole wheat couscous and whole grain cereals. Cereals should have at least 3 grams of dietary fiber per serving; breads should have minimum of 2 grams per slice.

Healthy whole grain cereal suggestions = Kashi Heart to Heart, Kashi Go Lean Crunch, Barbara's Shredded Spoonfuls, Barbara's Cinnamon Puffins, 100% Bran Flakes, General Mill's MultiChex, Oatmeal (unsweetened), Cheerios, Multigrain Cheerios.

2. Eat fresh or frozen fruit for dessert.

3. Choose cereals that have at least three grams of dietary fiber per serving.

4. Add beans to salads and soups, or have them as a side dish. Beans have more fiber than any other food (1/2 cup beans =

8 grams of dietary fiber). Try to have at least 1/2 cup of beans three times per week.

5. Snack on raw vegetables. Keep them cut-up in the fridge. Try hummus as a dip.

6. At lunch and dinner fill up on salad and vegetables. Vegetables and/or salad should cover at least half of your plate.

7. Make a fresh fruit smoothie. In a blender, add 1/2 cup skim or soy milk plus 1 cup fresh or frozen fruit (cut up) with a lot of ice. Blend and enjoy!

8. Make vegetables a main course such as vegetable chili, grilled vegetables or a veggie burrito. Add a side salad and a fruit.

9. Add a mixed greens salad to meals instead of a side of "mayonnaise-laden" macaroni salad, Cole slaw or French fries.

10. Add raw or grilled vegetables to your sandwiches.

Step 8. Eat Less Fat and Choose Them Wisely

Your best friend tells you to eat less fat. Your cousin slathers the butter on his bread and potatoes. Your uncle has high cholesterol and avoids fats altogether. Advice on fat seems to flip flop by the day.

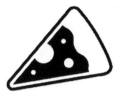

What gives?

For the past 30 years, fats have been blamed for everything from obesity to heart disease and cancer. Thankfully, new research shows that good fats, **in moderate amounts**, benefit your health. But we should all continue to lay off the bad fats that can increase the risk for heart disease. That's why it helps to **know your fats** in foods. Read on to become fat-savvy so you can make the right choices for your health and your weight.

Why do we need fat in our diets?

Yes, there are some "bad fats" to avoid. But there are so many reasons to get some good fats. Here are some of the benefits of eating fat:

-Provides and helps you absorb the fat-soluble vitamins, A, E, D and K.
-Helps make hormones you need to grow and develop.
-Gives you energy.
-Keeps you warm by providing insulation.
-Vital for beautiful hair and skin.
-Protects your organs.

Your body **requires** fat—but not as much fat as most people eat. When we talk about fat, a good place to start is with **cholesterol**.

What is cholesterol?

Cholesterol is a waxy substance found among fats circulating in your bloodstream and in all of your body's cells. Having some cholesterol in your body is needed for various functions, such as making vitamin D. However, high levels of cholesterol in your blood can lead to plaque in your arteries which may contribute to health problems such as heart disease and stroke.

Your body can make enough cholesterol on its' own. You do not have to consume it. The cholesterol-containing foods include meat, liver and other organ meats, poultry, fish, eggs, butter, cheese plus 2% and whole milk. The problem with these foods is not the cholesterol they contain, but the high amount of saturated fat some of them have. Fish, shellfish, eggs and skim and 1% milk are all low in saturated fat and in moderate amounts do not appear to increase blood cholesterol levels. On the other hand, this is another reason why plant foods are so healthy: you don't get any cholesterol or saturated fat (with the exception of palm and coconut oil) from plant foods.

These are the **four major factors** that can increase the amount of cholesterol in your blood, even if your dietary cholesterol intake is low:

-Eating saturated fats
-Eating trans fats
-Having extra body weight
-Not exercising

What is "good" and "bad" cholesterol?

When it comes to the cholesterol in your blood, doctors often talk about two types: One is "good" and one is "bad" for your health. The good cholesterol is HDL (short for "high-density lipoprotein") and the bad cholesterol is LDL (short for "low-density lipoprotein"). The list of major factors above can cause your LDL (the bad one!) levels to also increase and your HDL (the good one!) to decrease.

What are Triglycerides?

Triglyceride is another form of fat that's in your body. People who have high levels of triglyceride (>150 mg/dl) often have a low level of "good" cholesterol (HDL) and a high level of "bad" cholesterol (LDL). Triglyceride levels of 150 mg/dl or higher may increase your risk for heart disease. Many people with heart disease, diabetes or both, have high triglyceride levels. Triglycerides can be elevated if your diet is high in sugar and/or fat, if you are overweight or don't get enough exercise.

What are Dietary Fats?

These are the fats found in the foods you eat. They're the reason macaroni and cheese and rice pudding taste so creamy. Fats come naturally from a lot of foods: meat, poultry, fish, eggs, cheese, milk, oils, butter, nuts, and seeds. Fats are also added to foods like salad dressings, sauces, cookies, cakes, pies and fried foods.

Healthy vs. Unhealthy fats

You may know that some fats are considered "good" (healthy) or "bad" (unhealthy). To tell them apart, it helps to know the four groups of fats found in foods: saturated, trans, monounsaturated, and polyunsaturated. Fats in foods may contain a mixture of these four different kinds of fats. Read on for what they do and where you'll find them.

First, the two groups of "bad" fats, saturated and trans:

The Where and What on Saturated Fats

Where you get saturated fats
Saturated fats are found mostly in animal foods, such as red meats (beef, lamb, pork and veal), bacon, sausage, cheese, whole and 2% milk, cream and butter. Products, such as pizza and cookies, that include any of these ingredients, will also contain saturated

fat. Two vegetable oils, palm and coconut, are also rich sources of saturated fats.

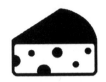

Saturated fats and your health

You don't need a certain amount of saturated fat in your diet. "Less is best" when it comes to eating saturated fats. For good health it's wise to keep your intake to 7% or less of your total calories. Eating saturated fats can **increase your risk** for coronary heart disease (CHD). In CHD the vessels that carry blood to your heart become clogged and don't work well. Eating less saturated fats and having "good" fats instead can lessen your risk for clogged arteries, help lower blood cholesterol (including LDL) and decrease the overall potential to develop heart disease.

The Where and What on Trans Fats

Where you get trans fats

Trans fats are liquid fats or oils that have hydrogen added to make them more solid. Food manufacturers add trans fats to foods so they don't spoil as quickly. If you see **partially hydrogenated, hydrogenated, or shortening** on a food label, it has trans fats. Trans fats are found in stick margarine, baked goods (such as crackers, donuts, cookies, croissants and pie crust), shortening and fried foods. You can keep your trans fat intake low by doing the following: choose tub margarines or–better yet–use olive oil, nut butter, hummus or avocado on bread, and avoid fried foods and baked goods that contain trans fats.

Trans fats and your health

Like saturated fats, trans fats can raise your blood cholesterol and LDL levels. For heart health, it is best to avoid them completely. If you see **partially hydrogenated or hydrogenated fat or shortening** on an ingredient list in the grocery store–leave it on the shelf or if it's in your pantry–throw it out! When the Nutrition Facts panel says the food contains "0 g" of *trans* fat, but it contains **any of the above three mentioned fats**, it means the food contains less than 0.5 grams of *trans* fat **per serving**. If you eat more than one serving, you could be getting a large dose of "artery-clogging" *tran fat.* Hopefully, trans fats will be banned soon. The good news is they're less common in packaged foods now since a 2006 law required U. S. food manufacturers to list them on the Nutrition Facts label.

Now, the two groups of "good" fats, monounsaturated and poly-unsaturated:

What are monounsaturated fats?

Where you get monounsaturated fats
These fats are sometimes called "Mediterranean" or heart-healthy. They are found in olives, olive oil, nuts, nut butter (peanut butter, almond butter, etc.), avocados, and canola oil. Try to eat these instead of saturated or trans fats whenever possible. For example, spread almond butter instead of regular butter on your toast.

Monounsaturated fats and your health
These fats are great for your health for so many reasons.

Look at all of these benefits monounsaturated fats provide:

-Lower your total cholesterol.
-Lower your bad (LDL) cholesterol.
-Raise your good (HDL) cholesterol.
-Lower your risk of heart disease and stroke.
-Provide Vitamin E, a vitamin that most people don't get enough of. Vitamin E is an antioxidant and is vital for keeping cells healthy.

What are polyunsaturated fats?

Where you get polyunsaturated fats

Vegetable oils, nuts and seeds are high in polyunsaturated fats. Eat these fats, along with monounsaturated fats, in place of saturated and trans fats. One way is to top your salad with a spoonful of sunflower seeds, slivered almonds or avocado slices instead of cheese.

Polyunsaturated fats and your health
Polyunsaturated fats can also help reduce the cholesterol levels in your blood and lower your risk of heart disease. They also include omega-3 "essential fats"—fats your body can't make and must get from food. Omega-3 fats (like those in salmon and walnuts) are important for brain function, growth, and development.

How much fat do we need per day?

Health experts recommend that teens, ages 15-19, get about 25 to 35 percent of their daily calories from fat. So if you're eating 1800 calories per day, 540 calories is ideal–that's 60 grams of fat. For 1500 calories, that is 50 grams of fat or 450 calories per day. You can figure it out by dividing the calories by nine, because each gram of fat gives you nine calories.

After you reach age 20, you need a little less: about 25% of your daily calories from fat. Staying within these amounts can reduce your risk for chronic diseases (like heart disease), while you still get enough of the nutrients in fat that you need.

Impact of fat calories on weight

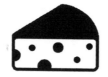

Fat is the most concentrated source of calories. At nine calories per gram, fat has more than double the calories of protein and carbohydrate (which have four calories per gram each). This explains why it's easy to add calories quickly to your meals when you eat high-fat foods.

Lets take a further look at how quickly fat calories can add up!

Let's analyze a salad rich in fruits and vegetables that you might choose at a restaurant. With two cups of spinach, 1/2 cup of sliced strawberries, a tablespoon of sliced almonds, and an ounce of goat cheese, it weighs in at a healthy 350 calories. But **add** on the four tablespoons (that comes on the salad) of dressing. Now you're looking at a 750-calorie salad! The four tablespoons of salad dressing can have more calories than the salad itself! So limit the dressing to two tablespoons (which is 200 calories), or better yet, use a tablespoon of olive oil and lemon or vinegar and save yourself an additional 100 calories! And, always, order the dressing on the side!

That's why paying attention to fat is a key strategy for losing weight and keeping it off. Keep tabs on foods high in fat, as well as added fats from French fries, sauces, butter, sour cream and salad dressing. It all adds up! If you can, check out the Nutrition Facts label for the serving size, calories per serving and amount of fat grams. **Just an FYI–five grams of fat equals one teaspoon of fat.**

How to choose healthy fats at home and when eating out
Fats from plants and fatty fish, such as salmon and tuna, are the best for us to eat. (The only plant fat exceptions are coconut and palm oils—they are high in saturated fat.) Healthy plant fats include avocado, nuts, nut butter, olives, olive oil, and canola oil. Try

to include one serving of these healthy plant fats with lunch and dinner. Use avocado in place of mayo or have an almond butter and strawberry sandwich instead of ham and cheese. If you eat fish, try to have fish as your protein choice at least twice a week. If you are going to eat meats and dairy products, go for the lower fat choices.

The following is a list of lower fat cuts of meat:
*Lean beef (round, sirloin, chuck, loin). Buy "choice" or "select" grades of beef rather than "prime."

*Lean or extra lean ground beef (no more than 15% fat).

*Lean veal (except commercially ground).

Lean ham, lean pork (tenderloin, loin chop). Ham and Canadian bacon are both low in fat but higher in sodium (salt) than other meats.

*Lean lamb (leg, arm, loin).

Here is the low fat dairy list:

Low fat dairy = skim or nonfat milk, 1% milk, 1% cottage cheese, nonfat yogurt, low fat cheese that contains 3 grams of fat or less per serving

Smart Tips for Eating Less Fat

1. Order salad dressing on the side. To use less, dip your fork into dressing and then into salad, instead of pouring it on.
2. Use hummus or avocado in place of mayonnaise on sandwiches.
3. Order a side salad, in place of fries, when dining out.
4. Measure oil with a measuring spoon, before you add it, when cooking.
5. Sauté vegetables in vegetable or chicken stock.
6. Limit full fat cheese to one slice or one ounce per sandwich.
7. Use olive oil, light margarine or whipped butter in place of stick margarine or butter.
8. Enjoy broiled, grilled or roasted foods instead of fried foods.
9. Avoid fatty meats such as bacon, sausage and pork ribs.
10. Limit red meat (beef, lamb, pork, and veal) to 3 ounces of cooked lean cuts to twice per week.
11. Use skim, 1% milk, soy, or almond milk in place of whole or 2% milk.
12. Choose low fat (2%) cheese in place of high-fat cheese.
13. Squeeze 1/2 lemon with 2 teaspoons of olive oil on your salad in place of bottled creamy dressing.

Step 9. Read Food Labels

Why should you read food labels?
I've had clients come to my office and tell me that they eat three cups of cereal for breakfast. So what? They didn't know a serving of cereal is usually about 3/4 to 1 cup. So often, we eat too much because we didn't check the label. For my clients eating cereal, reading the label would have saved them about 200 calories at breakfast (and a potential weight gain of about 20 pounds in one year!). It's not just about your cereal, though: Check out the label on the back of your favorite candy, granola bar, yogurt, salad dressing, bread, canned soup, tomato sauce, and more. If you want to lose weight, stay healthy, and maintain your new weight, reading food labels is a key skill to learn.

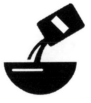

What else do you get from reading the food label?
Being aware of what you're consuming should make you a more mindful eater. You'll find out the calories, serving size, fiber, sugar, sodium, fat, ingredient list—and more. They are all important for keeping you healthy! If a food is not so healthy, such as a store-bought blueberry muffin, the info on the label can help you to either leave the product on the shelf or choose an appropriate serving size so it doesn't drive up your daily calorie intake. Read-

ing the Nutrition Facts label in the grocery store before you buy or in the kitchen as you prepare food puts you ahead of the game. Most people are clueless as to the number of calories they're consuming or how much they should be eating. You don't have to be. It's right there on the label. Just make sure you read it!

What can you learn from reading food labels?

The number one lesson to learn from food labels is **portion control**. This is what my clients who ate 3 cups of cereal needed to learn. The label will show you what a serving size is and how many calories are in each serving. It will also show you how many servings are in the package. If you plan to eat the entire package in one sitting, multiply the number of servings by the calories. Doing the math before you eat may just help you take a smaller portion. When it's time to eat, measure your portions with a measuring cup or spoons. In time you will see that you will be able to estimate a healthy portion size, which plays a big role in managing your weight.

The label also shows you the amount per serving of the three major nutrients (commonly known as macronutrients): protein, fat, and carbohydrate. They are broken down further under the headings of fat and carbohydrate. If you look at the label for fat grams, directly underneath you will see the breakdown for saturated fat, trans fat and cholesterol. The carbohydrate sections will be further divided into sugar and fiber grams.

Use the % Daily Values as Your Guide The % Daily Value (DV) shows the percentage of some key nutrients that come from one serving. The percentage is calculated for someone who follows a 2,000-calorie meal plan, but it's a good guide about how healthy a food is for everyone. If you want to consume **less** of an unhealthy nutrient (such as saturated fat, cholesterol or sodium), choose foods with a percent DV of 5% or less. If you want to consume **more** of a healthy nutrient (such as fiber or Vitamin C), choose foods with 20% DV or more.

What else does the label tell you?

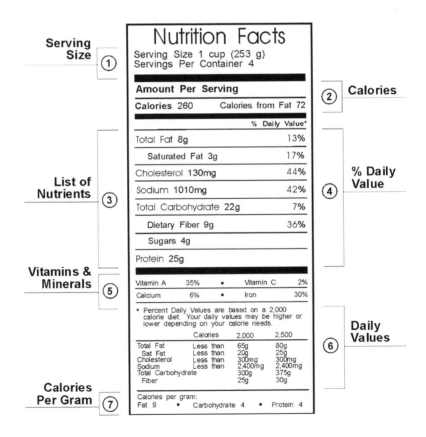

The Nutrition Facts food label is really a food's *best kept secret*. The label displays so much information that can help you make smart food choices. Here's what to look for:

Check label for **serving size** and **number of servings**.

Read calories per serving and **do the math** (#servings x calories), especially if you plan to eat more than one serving.

Check label for **fat grams**. Five grams of fat = 1 teaspoon of fat.

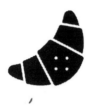

Look for **trans fats** on the Nutrition Facts label. There is no safe Daily Value (DV) for trans fats. Because trans fats are bad for your heart, if the product contains any, do your heart a favor and leave it on the shelf. Also read the **ingredient label** and look out for **partially hydrogenated or hydrogenated oil and/or shortening**. If you see any of these unhealthy fats, the product does, indeed, contain trans fats, so leave the product on the shelf! Just an FYI: When the Nutrition Facts panel says the food contains "0 g" of *trans* fat, but it contains any of the above trans fats, it means the food may contain up to 0.5 grams of *trans* fat **per serving**. Unfortunately, it can be listed as 0 grams as long as it is less than 0.5 grams per serving. So, if you eat more than one serving, you could be getting a large dose of "artery-clogging" *tran fat*.

Limit foods containing **saturated fat, cholesterol**, and **excessive sodium**. Choose foods that contain a Daily Value of 5% or less of these nutrients.

Check label for **sugar grams**. One teaspoon of sugar equals 4 grams. So if you divide the sugar grams by four, you will see how many teaspoons of sugar are in that particular food. Read the ingredient list for types of sugars. Sugar comes in many forms so look out for them on the label. Fructose, dextrose, corn syrup, honey and maple syrup are all types of sugar you may see on a label.

Make sure you **get 100% of these nutrients** each day: Vitamin A, Iron, Calcium, Vitamin C, and the B Vitamins: Thiamine, Riboflavin and Niacin.

Check the label for **fiber** grams. Whole grain (such as breads and cereals) or fruit/vegetable-based food products should contain at least three grams of fiber per serving.

Read the **ingredient list**. Ingredients are listed in descending order by weight. Those in the largest amounts are listed first. So the last ingredient is the smallest amount. In addition to possible trans fats, you want to pay attention to the types of sugars in the product. Although all sugars, no matter where they are derived from, are sugar, sugar from fresh fruit is healthier than corn syrup (aka dextrose). As for whole grains, if a product states it is a whole grain product, the first word on the ingredient list should be "whole." You may also want to avoid products with harmful colorings, additives and preservatives.

Below is an ingredient list from a box of oat cereal:

Ingredients:

Whole Grain Oats, Modified Corn Starch, Corn Starch, Sugar, Salt, Tocopherols, Trisodium Phosphate, Calcium Carbonate, Natural Colour. Contains Wheat Ingredients.

What do those nutrient claims mean on the product label?
Many packaged foods today also come along with nutrient content claims from the food manufacturer. You'll see them advertised on the front of a package. Luckily, these claims are overseen by the FDA and follow strict regulations.

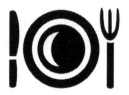

Health Claims on the Label

Read The Front of the Package

The front of the package is designed to grab your attention. Manufacturers use different packaging techniques to sell their products to us. For many years, health and nutrient content claims appeared on packages without any regulation. Today these claims, which include "high fiber," and "low fat," have standard definitions and requirements that you can use as a quick guide for making smart selections. By having some knowledge of the claims, you can more effectively and efficiently select foods and choose between products.

Health Claims

Health claims describe the link between a nutrient or a food and the risk of a disease. Products that make a health claim must contain a specific amount of the nutrient that is tied to the health-related condition.

For example, if a product is to make a claim about the relationship between sodium and hypertension (also known as high blood pressure), the product must not exceed 140 milligrams of sodium per serving. If the package states that the product "may reduce the risk of hypertension," we know that it is a low-sodium product, because low sodium is defined as 140 milligrams or less sodium per serving.

Additionally, the claims must make it clear that other factors, such as exercise or genetics, may also influence the development of certain diseases. Health claims cannot state the degree of risk reduction and must use words such as "may" or "might" in discussing the food-disease relationship. Examples of legitimate health claims on food labels include:

Fat and Cancer
Claim: A low-fat diet may help the risk for developing some types of cancer.
Requirements: 3 grams or less fat per serving or fish and meats that are "extra-lean" (fewer than 5 grams fat, fewer than 2 grams saturated fat, and fewer than 95 milligrams cholesterol per serving).

In addition to health claims on the Nutrition Facts label, many packaged foods today also come with **nutrient content claims** provided by the manufacturer. These claims are typically featured in ads for the foods or in the promotional copy on the food packages themselves. They are strictly enforced by the FDA.

The list below provides some of the most commonly used nutrient content claims along with the definition of the claim.
These claims are each based on **one serving.**

Calorie free = Less than 5 calories

Sugar free = Less than 0.5 grams of sugar

Fat free = Less than 0.5 grams of fat

Low fat = 3 grams of fat or less

Reduced fat or less fat = At least 25 percent less fat than the regular product

Lean = Less than 10 grams of fat, 4.5 grams of saturated fat and 95 milligrams of cholesterol

Extra lean = Less than 5 grams of fat, 2 grams of saturated fat and 95 milligrams of cholesterol.

Light (lite) = At least one-third less calories or no more than half the fat of the regular product, or no more than half the sodium of the regular product

Low cholesterol = 20 or fewer milligrams of cholesterol and 2 grams or less of saturated fat

Low sodium = 140 milligrams or less of sodium

Reduced or less sodium = At least 25 percent less sodium than the regular product

High fiber = 5 or more grams of fiber

Good source of fiber = 2.5 to 4.9 grams of fiber

You don't have to be a nutritionist or food scientist to understand the food label! To make label reading easy, here are some general guidelines.
If a product labels says:

"Free" = a food has the least possible amount of the specified nutrient.

"Very Low" and "Low" = the food has slightly more than foods labeled
"Free."

"Reduced" or "Less" = the food has 25 percent less of specific nutrient than the regular version of the food.

For more information on label reading, health claims and some of the widely used nutrient claims and what they mean: www.cfsan. fda.gov/label.html

Recommended app to use while grocery shopping: *Fooducate* (free for iPhone/Android) You can scan the package barcode with your phone to see if the **nutrition label** is living up to its merit and the product is truly healthy. If it's not, this app will give you suggestions for some healthier alternatives.

Step 10. Get Enough Sleep

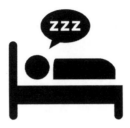

Sleep: What About It?

First comes school, sports, homework, jobs or more. You have so much to do just to get through the day—it's easy to see why sleep takes a backseat. Maybe you push yourself to stay up late. Or you get up early to start the next day. But how does it make you feel? Because sleep and well-being are tightly connected, not getting enough hours can make you feel irritable and make it hard to concentrate. By now, you've probably guessed what else skimping on sleep can do: It directly impacts your weight. We know from research that people who don't get enough sleep eat about 300 more calories per day and weigh more. If you're sleep deprived, you're more likely to make poorer food choices or brush off your exercise program. The last thing you feel like doing when you're tired is running around, right? And a chocolate fudge cookie will probably seem much more appealing than an apple! How many hours of sleep do you usually get? Studies show that **teens need 9 to 10 hours of sleep** per night. You're busy, but try to get the sleep you need to have energy, be active, lose weight, and feel healthy. And take advantage of the weekends to catch up on your sleep!

The Health Benefits of Sleep

It seems like you don't do much when you sleep. But many of your body's important activities happen while you're snoozing. That's why missing out on a few hours of sleep each night can cause so many problems. You need sleep to:

1. Repair your body tissues and promote their growth. During sleep you make growth hormone to promote development.
2. Lower your blood pressure.
3. Regulate the levels of hormones that affect your appetite.
4. Enhance your memory so you remember things—like the answers to your next test!
5. Decrease the amount of certain "stress hormones" (called cortisol and adrenaline). These hormones can add belly fat if they reach high levels.
6. Maintain your immune system. This explains why you're more likely to get sick and feel "run down" when you don't get enough sleep.

How Does Sleep Affect Weight?

Quite simply, being sleep-deprived makes you hungry. When you're low on sleep, you may just be eating to keep yourself wide awake. Researchers have found that your sleep-deprived body makes more of the hormone **ghrelin** and less of the hormone **leptin**. The problem is that ghrelin makes you feel hungry. Leptin, on the other hand, makes you feel full. Get 9 to 10 hours of sleep and you'll reap the benefits of leptin's fullness factor. You'll also skip more of the sedentary late-night TV watching and Internet surfing that prompt you to snack on unneeded calories.

Tips to Help You Sleep

1. A cup of chamomile tea before bed can help you relax and sleep.

2. Stop drinking caffeine and avoid chocolate after 6 p.m. Caffeine, in coffee, tea and chocolate, can affect your sleep, for up to 10 to 12 hours and wake you up during the night.

3. Avoid alcohol—it can also wake you up at night.

4. Limit food and beverage intake for three hours before bedtime to avoid indigestion. Drink more fluids during the day and stop drinking soon after dinner. Then you'll avoid the need to get up and go to the bathroom during the night.

5. Regular exercise is ideal but finish at least three hours before bed so you can relax.

6. Don't have a TV in the bedroom but reading for enjoyment is fine. This lets you keep your bedroom a place for quiet and rest.

7. If you feel stressed, practice stress management techniques, such as listening to music, positive self-talk, deep breathing exercises and yoga.

8. Avoid news about troubling events or intense video games just before bed so you feel relaxed.

9. A warm bath or shower right before bed may help you sleep.

PART 2

Conquering Different Eating Situations: Maintaining Your Weight and Healthy Lifestyle

Introduction

1. Overcoming Family and/or Peer Pressure to Sabotage Healthy Eating and Weight Loss Efforts

2. Vacations

3. Parties/Holidays

4. High school: Cafeteria Dining and Brown-Bagging Your Lunch

5. College: Living On and Off Campus

6. Restaurants

7. Fast Food

8. Late Night Eating

9. Managing Sugar Cravings

10. Overindulging On Any Occasion

Introduction

The typical American, over the age of eight, consumes at least four meals per week prepared in a commercial setting such as a restaurant or deli. Add on to that the meals consumed at school, friends' houses, parties and while on vacation, and you end up with a vast number of meals eaten outside the home. Because so many meals today are eaten away from home, learning how to make smart food choices is key to eating healthy and managing your weight. With a little planning, you can eat healthy wherever you go. Whether you're at a restaurant with friends, on vacation, at a holiday party or simply home alone at one in the morning watching a movie, you can learn the skills to manage your weight and eat well!

In this section you will explore ten different eating situations and encounter cutting-edge strategies to help you make the best food choices under any circumstance. Please use this section of the book to help you eat healthy and overcome life's obstacles whenever they get in your way. Also included are strategies you can use when family or friends try to steer you away from healthy eating. And remember–**sometimes**, even with the best intentions, we still don't always practice what we set out to do. The important thing to remember is to **get right back on track with your meal routine** at the next meal or snack. Life is not always perfect. Neither is eating! But you will find, trust me, that over time these healthy eating strategies will become part of your eating style. Wherever you are, you **can** make good food choices. What is important to know is that the choice is **yours**. By planning ahead you will succeed!

1. Overcoming Family and/or Peer Pressure to Sabotage Healthy Eating and Weight Loss Efforts

Although it is widely known that eating well and taking care of yourself go hand-in-hand, sometimes you may encounter pressure from friends (boyfriends and girlfriends included) or family members to not follow your healthy meal routine. They may tell you that you look great, are thin enough or you should **just** enjoy rich, sinful foods with the rest of them! But, of course, you know that **you** feel better and are happier when you stay on track by eating healthy, exercising and practicing self-care. So what can you do–and not start an argument!–to continue on your healthy path and not give in to their demands? Here are some tips to help you stay on the straight and narrow:

Alway stick with your meal routine. Eat every three to five hours. Not letting yourself get too hungry will help you to not overeat when you are with family or friends. Even if you do splurge on a dessert, it will be easier to have a small portion.

If you have friends or family members who are overweight, they may be unhappy now that you are changing your diet and losing weight. It is not that they don't want the best for you. It's just that they may want **you** to stay like them! For a variety of reasons some people don't like change, whether its moving to a new place, changing their usual diet or changing their body size. That is fine for them. But you know that eating well, exercising and having a healthy weight is the right thing for you. Explain to your family and friends that you know what **you** want and you plan to take care of yourself. Tell them you are not on a "diet."

You are trying to eat well so you will be healthier and safely lose weight. Tell them you respect how they live their lives, but you are doing what is healthy for you. If you parents seem concerned about your new way of eating, make an appointment with a Registered Dietitian (RD) who can review your diet and help ensure that it is nutritionally-sound. She/he can also determine what a healthy weight is for you. The RD can also reassure your parents that you are eating well.

Have a chat with your friends. Explain to them that you want to practice self-care by eating well, exercising and reaching a healthier weight. Tell them that it would make it a lot easier for you if they would not push you to eat the unhealthy foods that they like to eat. You still want to be friends and hang out with them. But you'd rather have some fruit, raw veggies or a granola bar than chips and dip. Don't let your food choices get in the way of friendship. If you want, share with them how you are feeling better. Maybe they will want to eat more like you!

2. Vacations

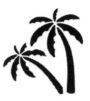

For some people, vacations are viewed as a time to kick off their shoes, let go of all restraints and indulge in those sinful foods they have been denying themselves. The real power of food is that it fuels and nourishes your body. You should remind yourself of this while on vacation when you are tempted to indulge in unhealthy foods or eat more than your body really needs. Malnutrition can result from overeating, just as it can result from under eating, so maintaining balance in your food choices is important to optimizing your *true* enjoyments in life.

So yes, vacations are meant to be a time to relax, enjoy new scenery and forget about the daily stressors of back-home living. Whether you are exploring an exotic location or trying an unfamiliar cuisine, all this can be accomplished while maintaining a healthy meal routine.   The food you eat should be healthy *and* enjoyable. Once you get to this realization, it *all* gets easier. You can have a great time on vacation, enjoy new and exciting food and all the while **not** gain weight. There are ways to eat healthy in every situation; it just takes a certain amount of knowledge, creativity and exploration.

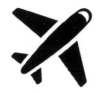

While you are on vacation, if you stay at a hotel and consume the majority of your meals in restaurants, you can still manage your weight. Set a goal for yourself before you go on vacation to **maintain your weight**. Do not worry about losing weight while you are away. Commit to yourself that you will enjoy yourself and still make smart choices. Practice mindful eating, make your choices selectively and watch your portion sizes.

If you are traveling to another country, take some time to research the area's cuisine and investigate the healthier options you might be interested in trying. Educate yourself about the culture and food you will experience. Many restaurants post their menu on the internet so check it out and prep yourself to ensure you make good choices.

Here are a few tips to keep in mind while you are traveling:

1. **Think before you eat.** This is an essential habit that you should develop in all situations which revolve around food.

2. **Eat in moderation.** You will be tempted with food you have never seen or rarely get to experience but make your choices selectively and stick to portion sizes. Since the variety of intriguing

food selections may increase while on vacation, cut back on the size of your typical meal and opt for a salad or vegetable soup and one appetizer instead. You will get to try a greater variety of food while having control over the total amount consumed for the day.

3. **Do not lose sight of your meal routine.** Start the day with a healthy breakfast. Request whole grain cereals and bread. Ask for skim or soymilk. Have fresh fruit if it's available. If you find that fresh fruit is limited on the menu, visit a local farmers' market or the local grocery store to pick up some fruit for snacks and dessert. Put emphasis on choosing vegetable or fish dishes and salads at lunch and dinner. Fresh fruit is a great choice for dessert. If you don't see fresh fruit listed on the menu, ask. Many dining establishments can put together a fresh fruit plate. If the restaurants only have rich desserts, have some fruit when you get back to your hotel room. Your meals should be nutritious; if you eat well, you will feel well. While on vacation you may be eating every meal out, so always think before you order.

Use the following meal suggestions to help you stay with your meal routine while on vacation:

*For breakfast: Eggs, unbuttered whole wheat toast and fresh fruit is a good choice. Whole grain cereal or oatmeal with skim, soy or other milk alternative, such as yogurt, and fresh fruit is another good option and one you will typically find on restaurant menus or hotel continental breakfasts. Always order your bread dry and, if you so desire, add butter or a small amount of jam. Be sure to limit the butter to one pat because each contains 100 calories and *that* is a small scoop of frozen yogurt! Keep in mind breakfast should contain servings from all the major food groups: whole grain, protein, low-fat dairy or non-dairy alternative and fruit and/

or vegetable. A healthy breakfast sets the stage for the rest of the day.

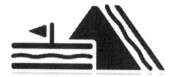

*As for lunch: sandwiches, broth-based soups and salads are often good options. Choose sandwiches that offer a source of protein such as grilled chicken, fish, or hummus on whole grain bread and go easy on the creamy condiments. Broth-based soups are healthier than cream-based so select the ones filled with vegetables and lean protein or beans. Choose salads that contain lean proteins such as grilled chicken, turkey, tofu, or beans; lots of veggies and healthy fat from nuts or seeds such as almonds, cashews, sunflower seeds or avocado and a vinaigrette dressing (served on the side) or a squeeze of fresh lemon.

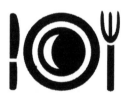

*Now for dinner: If you know you are going to a *fabulous* restaurant for dinner, have a light lunch. Or, if you opt for a more decadent lunch, go light on your choices at dinner while still trying a few different menu items. Also aim to increase your exercise on days when you know you may be eating a calorie-packed meal. Have a salad or broth-based soup as an appetizer and choose baked, broiled or grilled chicken or seafood as the main course paired with a vegetable side. Another option, order a few different appetizers to share as your meal. But avoid all fried appetizers as they are loaded in fat and calories. Keep the dessert light such as fresh fruit or share one dessert with everyone at the table. Sharing will help you maintain portion control and maintaining balance is the key to healthy living. These tips will ensure you stay on track and remain focused.

Aside from all the new and exciting food choices you might encounter while on vacation, since you are in a new place, take the time to explore! Be active: go walking, hiking, biking, swimming, or snorkeling. Welcome each day with a walk. You will feel invigorated and motivated to maintain your healthy lifestyle throughout the day. Seek out various tours that offer activities so you can learn and explore all at once. Take advantage of the hotel gym when the weather is not conducive to being outside. Keep in mind that vacation is not all about the food. Take the time to discover a new place and focus on the quality time spent with friends and family. In the end it is about the choices you make: the choices you make while you are on vacation and the choices you make every day at home. Aim to be your healthiest self!

Vacation Do's

1. Always keep to your meal routine.
2. Don't make food the focus of your trip. Enjoy your company and surroundings.
3. Be active! Talk long walks and become acquainted with the new locale. Rent a bike, swim (if someplace warm) or take a walking tour.

4. Visit a farmers' market or local grocery store to keep some fresh fruit on hand for snacks.
5. Bring a couple boxes of healthy granola bars with you when you travel. They're great for a mid-afternoon snack or when you are eating later than usual.
6. If you know you are going to eat a high calorie meal, be more active on that specific day.

3. Parties/Holidays

Quite often when you go to a party, healthy food is nowhere to be found. Piled on the table in sinful quantities are chips and dips, cookies and brownies and finger foods galore that could max out your calorie needs for the day with one plate-full! The drink options are typically soda or sugar- filled punches and teas that contain enough sugar to send your body soaring…only to plummet before the party has even begun. Is there any hope for me at this party you might ask? There is and it is all about your mindset and preparation. The best advice to help you avoid filling up on unhealthy party food: **don't go to the party hungry**. Make sure you eat before you venture out. That way you will not be hungry when you get there and will have much better control over what foods you do choose at the party. Take control and have a healthy meal before you leave your house. Going out on a full stomach will reduce your urge to eat the unhealthy, high calorie party food. It is always smart to plan ahead!

Let's explore five different meal options to eat before going out that will help you avoid overeating at the party:

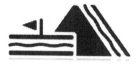

Option 1. Make a sandwich: Two tablespoons of peanut butter on whole grain bread is an easy, tasty and nutritious option. Try toasting the bread to melt the peanut butter for a slight alternative. The peanut butter contains healthy fats good for your heart and the whole grains will keep your energy from dipping. Add a cup of fresh fruit to satisfy your sweet tooth or slice up a banana, a handful of strawberries or an apple and add onto your sandwich.

Option 2. Have a cup of cereal: 1 cup of whole grain cereal plus 1 cup of skim milk, nonfat yogurt or milk alternative, such as soy or almond milk, and top with your favorite fruit. Whole grain cereals will list word phrases such as "whole grain" or "whole oats," as the first ingredient on the food label. Look for it. Keep the sugar content of the cereal below 10 grams per serving and the fiber should be at least 3 grams per serving.

Option 3. Open a can of soup: Enjoy a can of broth-based vegetable soup such as minestrone, lentil, vegetable barley, chicken vegetable or split pea. Look for soups with at least 4 grams of fiber and 140 calories or less per serving. Have a serving of fresh fruit along with the soup. The fiber and fluid should keep you going for several hours. Put your dancing shoes on and have fun!

Option 4: Make a smoothie: 1/2 cup vanilla or plain yogurt or soy or skim milk, 1 small banana and a cup of ice. This is your base recipe and is delicious as is. If you desire, add in one of the following: ½ cup of your favorite fruit such as blueberries or strawberries and/ or one tablespoon of peanut butter. Blend in blender and enjoy!

Option 5: Build a burrito: Into a microwave safe bowl add ½ cup black beans or ½ cup fat free refried beans plus 1 oz. low fat shredded cheese. Heat mixture in microwave for 30 seconds. Serve on a whole wheat tortilla wrap and top with 2 heaping spoonfuls of salsa. This will satisfy your salty taste buds and steer you away from the chips and dips at the party.

But there will always be those times when, for some reason or other, you can't eat before you go out. It is life. It happens! **For emergencies:** keep a couple healthy granola bars with you. One to two granola bars, such as Kashi TLC, Lara, Cliff or Kind, can keep you full for a few hours. They're great to keep on hand (but please limit to no more than two granola bars per day!). If all fails and you are hungry when you arrive at the party, all is not lost! If you have a game plan you can still **practice moderation** in your food choices.

So, here you are at the party. What are you to eat when the majority of the options in front of you would quickly sabotage any intentions you had to eat healthfully?

The following tips will help you view parties as fun times with friends rather than an excuse or opportunity to eat junk food:

1. First, search for nutritious options. Peanuts, almonds or any nut-mixture will be chock-full of healthy fats that will keep you

satisfied longer than the icing on that cupcake. Just keep in mind when you are reaching for the nuts, the amount you grab should be about one handful.

2. Scan the dips and opt for salsa or any bean dip. Steer clear of the creamy, cheesy dips because, characteristically, these contain high amounts of saturated fat and calories. Portion out one handful of chips and pile on the salsa.

3. If by chance, fruits and vegetables are offered, by all means, fill your plate. But, just like the chip dips, be mindful of the veggie and fruit dips. Ranch and blue cheese dressing easily packs in 200 calories and 15 grams of fat in just 2 tablespoons and those sweet dips; well they can contain the equivalent of three sugar packets in just 2 tablespoons. Try to make a little go a long way and get your fill by eating more veggies.

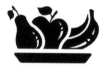

Now, the situation may very well be that **NONE** of the aforementioned options are available. **So what are your options now? Use the following tips to keep you on track!**

- If you are feeling hungry, scan the choices and select a couple foods you really like and perhaps do not get to eat often; take a reasonable amount and enjoy. Just remember, one serving, one trip. Finger foods are just that, foods to be eaten moderately while in conversation with others; they should not be the importance of your time at the party.
- Drinking water or seltzer at the party will also help keep you feeling full.
- By choosing a few of your favorites, your cravings will be satisfied without spearheading a tumble into a food coma!
- Focus on your friends and family. You will get more enjoyment out of laughing with those who are closest to you than indulging in unhealthy party foods. Do not let the food table become your focus.

4. High School: Buying Lunch at School

While it is always a good decision to bring a healthy lunch from home, sometimes you may not have the time or food available. So, off to school you go without a lunch. But you don't have to starve! You can find good options in the school cafeteria; you just have to know what to look for. Avoid giving in to temptation by the fries, cookies and chips dangling in front of you as you go through the line. You will be in better shape if you stick to the school lunch line rather than venture over to the vending machines. You will most likely find a vegetable and fruit offering as well as a suitable entrée. Be smart with your condiment choices as they can easily pile on unwanted saturated fat. In general, creamy condiments such as mayonnaise and ranch dressing will contain significantly higher amounts of fat than mustard, ketchup, hot sauce or salsa. Take a smaller plate, if available at the beginning of the lunch line, as it will help you to eat less.

Here are some healthy meal suggestions:

1. If you choose pizza, have one cheese slice and pair it with a salad, vegetable and/or a piece of fruit. Pizza is fine, if you stick to **one** slice. But avoid pizza that is loaded down with cheese

and piled high with various meat toppings, such as pepperoni. Choose healthier toppings, if available, such as mushrooms, onions, spinach and peppers.

2. Scope out the sandwich choices and opt for grilled chicken, turkey or ham and remember to watch how you "dress" the sandwich. Ask for whole grain sliced bread over white rolls and bread. Pile the sandwich with lettuce and tomato. Mustard is a healthier choice than mayonnaise.

3. Salad that includes some protein is another nutritious option. Chickpeas, hard-boiled eggs, nuts, grilled chicken or canned tuna are healthy proteins that will fuel your body for several hours. And you can have unlimited amounts of non-starchy vegetables in your salad. Ask for the dressing on the side so you can control the amount. Keep in mind vinaigrettes are typically better than the creamy stuff but either way, keep it to two tablespoons.

4. As far as beverage selection, water is **always** the best choice. Water is what your body needs to stay hydrated. Bring a stainless-steel thermos filled with water from home.

High School: Brown-Bagging Your Lunch

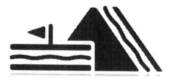

You will most likely find it is easier to pack a nutritious lunch than choosing something healthy from school. Aim to pack your lunch at least three times each week. If you know you are usually strapped for time in the morning, **pack your lunch the night before.** Eating the right combination of foods throughout the day will help keep you energized, focused and full. Your energy level will stay constant and you will feel most confident because you know you are feeding your body what it needs. In turn you're ensuring yourself that you are taking good care of your body. Just keep in mind that you want it to be healthy, tasty and portable. A packed lunch may seem boring, but you can make it nutritious *and* delicious. With a little effort, variety, spice and creativity you may find you actually enjoy your brown-bagged lunch.

Try these strategies to help you make a healthy lunch:

1. **Choose sandwich or main food item**:

*Peanut butter (or other nut butter) on whole grain bread. For an alternative to jam, add several slices of whole fruit such as banana, strawberries, kiwi or apple slices. Limit the peanut butter to two tablespoons per sandwich. You can also freeze a bunch of peanut butter sandwiches in advance in individual baggies. Grab one on the way to school and it will be defrosted and ready to eat by lunchtime.

*Chicken or tuna salad in a whole grain pita wrap.Ingredients for one serving: 1 (3 ounce) can of chicken or tuna, 1 diced celery stick, ¼ cup diced apples or sliced grapes. For the dressing: 1 tsp. olive oil, 1 tsp. Dijon mustard, 1 tsp. honey, 2 tsp. lemon juice.

*Egg salad on whole wheat bread. Ingredients for one serving of egg salad: 1 boiled egg (chopped), 1 tsp. mayonnaise, 1 tsp. Dijon mustard, 1 tsp. paprika, 1 Tb. diced onion, pepper. Mix together. Put on two slices whole grain bread with lettuce and tomato.

*Salad. Build it. Start with your greens (such as spinach, arugula, romaine or red leaf), add in any raw vegetable(s) you so desire (cucumber, grape tomatoes, red pepper, carrots, broccoli and/or cauliflower), add in a protein (2 hard-boiled eggs or 2 ounces low fat cheese or 3 ounces tuna or 1/2 cup black beans or chickpeas or 6 ounces tofu), add in healthy fat (1 tbsp. mixed nuts, sunflower seeds, or 1/4 avocado) and dress it (1 to 2 tbsp. vinaigrette or light dressing). Make enough for a few days and pack it in a Tupperware.

2. **Add one snack item**: Pre-packaged snacks such as a granola bar, string cheese or nonfat yogurt. Or portion out one serving size of trail mix (2 ounces), popcorn, air-popped (3 cups) or mixed nuts (1 ounce).

3. **Add fruit and/or vegetables**: Wash and cut-up fresh peppers, carrots, cucumbers, celery, broccoli or cauliflower. Separate into baggies to have for the week. In a Tupperware container, portion out 2 tablespoons of hummus, guacamole, or low fat salad dressing. Or simply bring a fresh fruit, such as an orange, apple or banana.

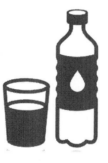

4. **Add a drink**: Water, always water: pack bottled water or, ideally, fill a thermos or sports bottle with filtered tap water from home.

Snacks for after school are important, too! Here are a few tips:

1. If you have after-school activities or sports, it's smart to keep a couple granola bars in your backpack at all times in case you forget to grab something in the morning on your way out the door.

2. If you have the time, include a snack such as a fruit paired with a small handful of nuts or a healthy granola bar and a cheese stick. Combining a healthy complex carbohydrate such as a fruit or a cup of whole grain cereal with a protein, such as a cheese stick or a small handful of nuts, will hold you over until dinner.

3. If you are playing an endurance sport you may want to pack a peanut or almond butter sandwich and fresh fruit to keep you well-fueled. Always keep a sports bottle filled with water to stay hydrated.

5. College Eating

Going to college is a major life change as well as a stepping-stone into adulthood. With this newfound independency comes responsibility. You are now in charge of everything you choose to eat, so arming yourself with the knowledge of healthy eating is one of the best things you can do for your body. Making good choices for your health will create a domino effect into other aspects of your life.

Whether you are living at home or hundreds of miles away, in college you will be faced with more decisions than you have ever before had in your life. Making food choices is just one of them, but one of the most important! Always aim to be mindful of what you choose to eat. Instead of consuming the majority of your meals at home you will now be eating in the college cafeteria, cooking in your own apartment, or stopping into local diners or fast-food joints for a quick bite to eat. Either way, it will be your choice, every day and every meal. College will keep you busy; it is a hectic yet exciting time and your schedule will be like no other you've ever had in the past or will likely have in the future. College life is unique but while the variability of every day is exciting, it often leaves you little time to worry about what to eat. You may have class during the lunch hour, a group project to work on well into dinnertime, or a work schedule that prevents you from eating at your "normal" times. Taking the time to plan your meals becomes ever more important. With a small amount of preparation and good choices you can maintain a healthy weight, and even lose weight, while in college. Let's take a look at how you can practice your healthy eating skills while in college, whether living on or off campus.

Living on Campus

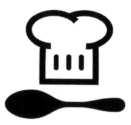

The major problem with college dining halls is the numerous food options that are offered in unlimited quantities, all equally intriguing and tempting. Faced with so many choices you, starved and heads-pinning, unable to make a decision, pile four strikingly different foods onto your plate. When else did you have the option of eating fried chicken, a burrito and plate of spaghetti plus unlimited desserts (!) all in one sitting? Having all these food options at your reach with the mere swipe of the school ID is what leads to the ever so prevalent, not so popular, **freshman 15**.

To keep you on track so you do not return home for Christmas break with extra weight, you need to be mindful of your choices and portion sizes. It is important to stick to your meal routine as much as possible. Read these tips carefully!

Tip #1: Don't skip breakfast or you will be ravenous come lunch time. If you don't have time to sit down and eat breakfast, bring a couple of healthy granola bars (such as Kashi TLC, Lara or Kind) along with you and eat them on the way to, or during, class.

Tip #2: If you know ahead of time you won't be eating dinner until late, have a healthy snack between 3:00 and 4:00 PM to curb your hunger. Keep some granola bars or a yogurt, dried fruit or fresh fruit or 100-calorie bag of popcorn on hand for a quick snack. Starving yourself at any point in the day is never effective when trying to lose weight or even maintain weight. Stick with your meal routine throughout the day to keep your hunger level low and energy level up.

Tip #3: If your schedule is hectic, it may be a good idea to have 5 or 6 small meals and snacks throughout the day. Keep healthy food options on hand in your dorm and in your backpack in case you can't make it to the cafeteria.

For a quick breakfast, a few good options include:

1. Instant unsweetened oatmeal, a handful (10 to 20) of almonds and a fruit. Add one teaspoon of sugar or stevia if you want some sweetness.

2. Make a yogurt parfait: 1/4 cup low fat granola, a cup of low fat yogurt and a fruit.

3. 1 cup low sugar cereal (such as Cheerios or Barbara's Cinnamon Puffins) plus 1 cup skim, soy or almond milk, a small handful of nuts and a fruit.

For a quick snack, options include:
*1 granola bar or nuts (10 to 20) and 1 fruit
*100-calorie pack popcorn and nuts (10 to 20)

*raw vegetables, such as cucumbers or carrots, and hummus (4 tbsp.)

*a string cheese and fruit, fresh or dried

*1 tbsp. peanut butter on whole grain crackers (4), a whole grain sandwich thin plus an apple

For lunch (if you are eating in the cafeteria) healthy suggestions include:

1. Vegetable soup (broth-based) and salad with grilled chicken or beans. Have a small whole grain roll and fresh fruit.

2. Grilled chicken, turkey sandwich, veggie burger or peanut butter sandwich. Request whole grain bread instead of a roll. Lettuce and tomato on the sandwich will help keep you full longer. Mustard, avocado, ketchup, barbeque sauce or pesto are healthier than mayonnaise, Add a side salad (avoid the fries!) and fresh fruit for dessert.

Dinner suggestions include:

1. Salad, grilled chicken or fish, vegetables and a small amount of brown rice, beans or baked potato. Remember: At least 1/2 of your plate should be vegetables.

2. Whole grain pasta with vegetables. Have tomato sauce or garlic and olive oil. Avoid rich sauces such as Alfredo. Ask for a small scoop of pasta (one cup is a good amount!) and a lot of vegetables. Add a salad and fresh fruit.

3. Vegetarian chili, stir-fry vegetables with tofu and/or chicken or vegetable/bean soup with a side of sauteed or grilled veggies and a salad. Have fresh fruit for dessert.

Living off Campus

One of the great things about living off campus is having access to your own kitchen. This gives you greater control over what food you shop for and choose to consume. **Make a conscious effort to stick with your meal routine.** More times than none, you can cook a healthier meal for yourself than you could choose from the school cafeteria.

Stay stocked with the basics from this extensive list and shop weekly for fresh foods such as fruits, vegetables, fresh meats, milk/milk alternative, yogurt and eggs. Avoid purchasing too many prepackaged processed foods; these will increase your food cost and provide much less nutritional value for your buck. You can create some great meals with these basics. Refer to the sample meal plan, meal ideas and one-week menu in Part 3. Tools of the Trade for meal suggestions.

To ensure you'll cook most of your meals at home, stock your kitchen with the following necessities:

<u>Basic Cookware</u>

A good knife and cutting board

Spatula

8" and 14" skillet with lid

Deep baking dish

Blender

<u>Food basics</u>

Spices such as garlic powder, oregano, rosemary, basil, red pepper flakes, ginger, chili pepper, thyme, cumin, curry, cayenne

Salt and pepper

Oil mister

Olive and/or canola oil

Balsamic vinegar

Vegetable or chicken broth

Tomato sauce

Condiments such as mustard, ketchup, soy sauce, pesto

Frozen vegetables (plain–without sauce; great with pasta or as side dish)

Frozen meals for when you don't have time to cook (Amy's, Kashi and Lean Cuisine are all good options)

Canned soups (great for lunch, dinner or snack–Amy's and Health Valley are healthy options)

Ready-to-eat whole grain/low sugar cereals (such as Cheerios--Plain or Multigrain–and Barbara's Cinnamon Puffins)

Oatmeal packets (unsweetened)

Whole grain bread/sandwich thins(can keep several loaves frozen for later use)

Whole grain pasta, rice, couscous and quinoa

Black beans, cannellini, kidney, lentils and chickpeas (same as garbanzo beans). FYI: rinse canned beans with water to get rid of some of the sodium. Veggie burgers-Dr. Praegers, Morningstar Farms and Amy's are great choices for a quick-and-healthy meal

Explore websites, such as www.myrecipes.com or download apps, such as SparkRecipes, that provide healthy recipes. Recipes are also included at the end of Part 3. Tools of the Trade. You will find you can cook to your tastes without having to add in all the fancy extras. Keep it simple, tasty and healthy. Always have several healthy granola bars with you (limit to two bars per day) in case you go to the library or have to stay late at school and can't get home to eat at your usual time.

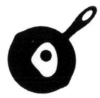

Take-Away Message:

1. Stay stocked with these basics and shop weekly for fresh foods such as fruits, vegetables, fresh meats, milk/milk alternative, yogurt and eggs.

2. Avoid purchasing too many pre-packaged processed foods; these will increase your food cost and provide much less nutritional value for your buck. You can create some great meals with the basics.

3. Refer to the sample meal plan, one-week menu and meal ideas in this book for suggestions. Explore websites, such as www.myrecipes.com or download apps, such as SparkRecipes, that provide healthy recipes (and don't forget the recipes included in Part 3. Tools of the Trade).

4. Always have several granola bars (limit to two per day) with you in case you go to the library or have to stay late at school and can't get home to eat at your usual time.

6. Restaurants

Over 30% of meals in the US are consumed at restaurants or on the run and it looks like this trend is here to stay. Between grabbing lunch from a food cart and socializing with friends at a restaurant, eating out has become so integrated into our daily lives. The good news is we don't necessarily have to give it *all* up in order to be healthy. Due to the increased public awareness regarding our *state of poor health*, restaurants have responded to the pressure by offering healthier choices and now, on almost every menu in America you can find a suitably healthy offering. Becoming savvy about ordering your meals is an extremely useful skill. It's all in your hands–the knife and fork! Learning how to single out the healthier options on the restaurant menu with a quick glance will serve you well, now and in the future.

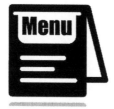

Before even stepping into the restaurant, familiarize yourself with the menu to have an idea of what you plan to order. Most restaurants, even food carts, have their menus listed on the web. If you do not see anything on the menu you would classify as considerably healthy, chose another restaurant if it's in your control. There are plenty of restaurants out there with healthy selections. Be conscious of portion sizes and educate yourself as to how the food is prepared.

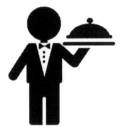

Here are some strategies to help you eat smart when dining out:

1. Avoid consuming the ever-so-large portion. Quite often restaurants serve entrees large enough to feed three or four people. If, when your food is served, you notice the copious amount is more than enough for one, kindly ask the waiter for a container to pack-up half and save for another meal. Or, if you are eco-conscious, bring your own reusable container from home.

2. Share an entree with your friend and get a salad as an appetizer. You could also order a salad as the first course and a healthy, non-fried appetizer as the entree. These strategies are also pocketbook-friendly and will leave you feeling satisfied.

3. When looking over the menu seek out healthy low fat choices. Salads *can* be a healthy option, but if you aren't careful, they can amount to more than a thousand calories. These heftier salads often contain components such as cheddar or Monterey

jack cheese, deli meats, nuts, bacon, dried fruit, croutons and creamy dressing. One or two of these components will not make your salad equivalent to a Big Mac, but having *several* fat and protein toppings most certainly will. More times than none, you can modify salads on menus. Here are some "tried and true" tips for ordering a lower calorie salad:

-Request a few of the heftier toppings, such as cheese and bacon, be removed and add in more vegetables such as roasted red peppers, artichokes, olives, or black beans if you see these listed anywhere else on the menu. If you don't see them listed, ask. They often have them!

-If you are a cheese person, have it as your protein source, or ask for it on the side and use a small amount. Feta and blue cheese offer more flavor in a much smaller portion than cheddar.

-Ask for the salad dressing on the side as well and keep in mind vinaigrettes are the heart-healthy choice. Balsamic vinegar or lemon plus olive oil is one of the best options. Limit it to two spoonfuls worth and you will save hundreds of calories. Creamy dressings often contain 200+ calories for only two tablespoons.

4. Other suitable entrée choices include grilled chicken or fish paired with vegetables and a small potato, rice pilaf or other healthy starch option. In general, grilled or baked is better than pan-seared or fried. Most restaurants allow you to substitute for different sides so make your choices wisely. Allow yourself one starchy side and have the other in the form of a vegetable. If a dish comes with a sauce, order it on the side.

5. Cream and cheese sauces are generally much higher in fat and calories than marinara.

6. For drink options, stick to water, seltzer or unsweetened iced tea or coffee.

7. If craving dessert, order fresh fruit. If you desire something richer, share with a friend.

As you can see there are many ways to make healthy choices at a restaurant. By making smart choices you will be able to manage your weight plus feel and look great! Here is a "snapshot guide" to assist you in making the healthiest choices when eating out, whether you go to an ethnic restaurant, a town pub or your local diner.

Traditional American and Ethnic Cuisines: The Good and The Not-So-Good

Cuisine	Healthy Choices	Foods to Avoid
American	Grilled chicken or veggie burger on whole grain bread, Grilled/baked chicken, fish or pork, broth based soup and salad, Sirloin steak	French fries, cream soups, fried chicken, fried fish, cheesy or casserole-like sides, fried sandwiches, loaded baked potato
Italian	Minestrone soup and salad, Mussels, Margarita Pizza, Grilled fish Chicken or Veal Marsala, Spaghetti with tomato sauce, Pasta Primavera, Salmon and Roasted Potatoes, Pasta with chicken or seafood (Note: request whole wheat pasta)	Shrimp Alfredo Pasta, Stromboli, Calzone, Manicotti, Lasagna Bolognese, Cheese or Beef Ravioli, Chicken Parmesan, Penne ala Vodka, Baked Ziti, Pepperoni or pasta on Pizza

Chinese	Seafood soup, Steamed Vegetables, brown rice, dishes that are Jum (poached), Chu (broiled), Kow (roasted) or Shu (barbequed), Shrimp or chicken with broccoli, Mixed Vegetables, Vegetable soup, Egg drop soup, Tofu with Mushrooms, brown rice	Won ton soup, Fried rice, Egg rolls, Lo Mein, Chow fun, Spare ribs, General Tsao's chicken, Crispy beef, Sweet and Sour Pork
Japanese	Tofu and vegetable soup, seafood soup, miso soup, edamame, seaweed salad, grilled, steamed or roasted plates (upon request), yakitori, sashimi, crab and avocado sushi roll, sushi (ask for cucumber in place of rice), Teriyaki with salmon, tofu or chicken.	Tempura, fried dumplings, donburi (fried pork), fried sushi rolls, sushi with spicy mayo or cream cheese
Greek	Hummus with pita, baba ghanoush, Tzatziki (limit to 2 tbsp.), potatoes, Greek salad with dressing on the side, chicken souvlaki, grilled octopus, lamb or fish with steamed vegetables, bean salad	Fried calamari, fried fish

| Mexican | Gazpacho, black bean soup, salsa, pico de gallo,tamales, guaca-mole, chicken, shrimp or vegetable fajitas, grilled chicken or sea-food soft tacos, bean burrito, pollo al car-bon, salad with grilled shrimp or chicken | Chips, Nachos, taco salad, sour cream, chi-michangas, quesadillas, sopapillas (fried pastry), enchilada platter |

You can eat sensibly and cut calories when eating out by selecting alternatives from "the usual" that are lower in fat and sugar. If the healthy alternatives are not listed on the menu, simply ask your server if they can prepare something "**special request**."

Try these healthy swaps:

Swap these:	For these:
Cream soups	Broth-based soups with vegeta-bles and/or beans
Buffalo chicken wings	Peel-and-eat shrimp
Quiche and salad	Broth-based soup and salad
Cornbread, muffins and rolls	Whole grain bread and small whole grain rolls
Fried chicken sandwich	Grilled chicken sandwich
Hamburger on white bun	Veggie burger or grilled porto-bello mushroom sandwich on whole grain toast
French fries	Side salad, baked potato, steamed or sauteed veggies
Creamy coleslaw	Tossed salad or sauteed/grilled/steamed veggies
Ice cream	Fresh fruit or sorbet

Restaurant Do's

1. Take the time to review the menu before you order. Most restaurants have their menus on the internet so you can make healthy choices before you go.

2. Make special requests to ensure that your meal is healthy.

3. Start your meal with a garden salad or a bowl of broth-based vegetable soup.

4. Order salad dressing on the side. Vinaigrettes are usually the best dressing choice. Dip your fork into the dressing and then into the salad. This will minimize your intake of dressing.

5. Ask for whole grain or rye sliced bread if ordering a sandwich. Avoid hefty white rolls, bagels and large sandwich buns. And you can always ask your server to take away the breadbasket if you want!

6. If you use butter for your bread, limit to one pat.

7. Order meats, chicken or fish grilled.

8. If there is a sauce served with your entree, request it on the side.

9. If you have a baked potato, omit the sour cream or have it served on the side and use one tablespoon or less.

10. If you would like dessert, order fresh fruit (they usually have it even if not listed on the menu!) or share one dessert with your companion(s).

7. Eating in Fast Food Restaurants

Truth be told, fast food is not the healthiest choice. However, when time is tight and you need a quick meal or you want to socialize with friends and the only place they want to go to is a fast food joint, chances are you will at some point find yourself placing an order at such a place. The good news is most fast food restaurants offer acceptable selections that can fit into your healthy eating plan; you just need to know what to look for and how to order.

Follow these healthy tips when making your fast-food order and you will be fine. As I said before, if you do some planning in advance **you can eat healthy anywhere!**

1. Before you go, look over the nutritional content of fast-food items by visiting the chain's website to identify the healthiest choices. Some chains also post their nutritional information near the counter or provide it in pamphlet form, but it is best to prepare before you visit.

2. If you have an iPhone, download the (free) app **Fast Food Calories**. This is a great app that provides the nutrition information for more than 100 fast food and sit-down chains. **Calorie**

King is another amazing (and free!) iPhone app that contains menu information.

3. Take a pass on the "super-size" option. These offers attempt to sway you to spend more money by offering a larger portion of really cheap food items such as fries and sodas. Know that you are not getting anything, nutrient-wise, for this extra cost to your pocket book. These larger portions will only increase your waistline!

4. Change out your side. Instead of fries order a healthier side dish such as a side salad or fruit cup.

5. Choose grilled chicken sandwiches or veggie burgers without sauce– both are a much healthier option than fried chicken or fish and are typically leaner than most burgers. By ordering grilled, broiled or baked you will save yourself over 100 calories.

6. Avoid ordering sandwiches with double meat. A single serving of meat is 2–3 ounces or about the size of a deck of cards. One meat patty alone is greater than this single serving size, so no need for the extra patty.

7. Avoid adding bacon to sandwiches because it is high in saturated fat, sodium and calories and offers very few nutrients. Instead, load your sandwich up with pickles, onions, lettuce, tomatoes, mustard and ketchup as all of these options are low in calories. These toppings will provide a little crunch to your meal and will be kind to your waistline.

8. Request whole wheat, pumpernickel or rye toast in place of a white bun, roll or wrap if this is an option. If only a white bun or wrap, eat just half.

9. Choose your condiments wisely. Hold the mayonnaise and other calorie-laden sauces and dressings. "Special sauce" is typically code for "full-of-fat" so go without or ask for it on the side to control how much you use. Mustard, ketchup, hot sauce or barbeque sauce are much better condiment choices.

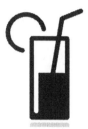

10. As for beverages, order water, seltzer, skim milk or unsweetened iced tea. If you want a little sweetness in your tea, add one packet of sugar or stevia. If you like stevia, keep a few packets with you.

It the right options are chosen, fast food can **occasionally** fit into you meal routine. However, fast food as a whole should be consumed in limited amounts as *all* of it is packed-full of preservatives, sodium, and numerous ingredients you cannot pronounce. If consumed regularly, you will possibly deprive your body of valuable nutrients you could easily acquire from healthy whole foods. You may also find that you don't feel well, may be lacking in energy or have difficulty concentrating in school. Take the time to nourish yourself. If at least 80% of your meals are from healthy whole foods, you are doing well. **Balance is key**.

8. Late Night Eating

Late night eating can be an obstacle for many teens in their efforts to either lose weight or maintain a healthy weight. However, there are several techniques you can use to avoid this. Additional pounds can quickly tack on if late night snacking is habitual, so if you find yourself munching in the wee hours of the night more than twice a month, you may need to reign in your habits. If you see it becoming a regular pattern it's time to figure out why you are eating late and get to the root of the problem. First think about why your late night snacking occurs. Some of the most common reasons are: 1) you skipped dinner; 2) stayed up late stressing over a project or exam; 3) drank too much alcohol (Remember: the legal drinking age in the U.S is 21); 4) were around friends who were also eating late at night; 5) or have formed a habit of it. Figure out your reason and let's discuss ways to overcome:

1. **If you skipped dinner**, you may need to reinforce your meal routine. Ensure you eat enough at dinner to help avoid snacking late at night. Go back to the basics and make sure your dinner is a healthy one.

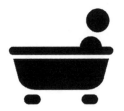

2. **If you are feeling stressed**, find alternative ways to relieve your anxiety. Food will only feed the stress. Enjoy a relaxing bubble bath or shower, listen to a few favorite songs or settle down with a good book.. Drinking a cup of decaffeinated herbal tea, such as chamomile, may also help you unwind and relax.

3. **If you drank too much alcohol** (Remember: the legal drinking age is 21 in the U.S.), you may ultimately need to ask yourself why you drank so much. Eating a decent meal before having a drink may help prevent late night eating. Alcohol can lower your blood sugar which leads to feeling hungry and, thus, weight gain. **Always** keep in mind you should never drink to the point of not being able to control yourself.

4. **If you are frequently around friends who indulge in late night eating**, continue to hang out with them if you like. But if you aren't hungry, **don't eat**. Have water or seltzer. If you go to a diner with your friends and don't want to feel like a "party-pooper," order fruit. Grapefruit, cantaloupe and fresh fruit salad are usually available in late night eating spots. Or go home and get some sleep!

5. If you find you are actually hungry at night, opt for a snack that is both filling and low in calories. What you want to go for are foods that are high in fiber and low in sugar. Some options include a bowl of vegetable soup, a cup of high fiber cereal with skim or soy milk, a serving of fresh fruit, two rice cakes each topped with a teaspoon of nut butter, raw vegetables and hummus or a 100-calorie bag of popcorn. Portion out your servings and **eat mindfully**!

6. If late night eating has become a habit, recognize you *can* break it. Make sure you eat enough throughout the day when you are most active and **halt** the late night eating cycle. Try not to eat after dinner or limit yourself to herbal tea, fruit or a granola bar. It may take three nights of not eating after dinner for your body to get used to it. Breaking an unhealthy habit is never easy but with practice and determination it can be done. Keep in mind your motivation and never lose sight of your goal.

9. Managing Sugar Cravings

For most of us when we get a craving, it's for sugar. Whether for a quick "pick-me-up," a mid-afternoon treat, a late-night indulgence or (for girls!) that time of the month, something sweet surely makes the top of the list! Even at birth, babies prefer the taste of sweet over any other. Why so, you ask? Sugar stimulates the release of the body's "feel good chemical" serotonin, which calms and relaxes us. However, after eating the bag of jelly beans, this feeling of immense pleasure quickly plummets along with your blood sugar. And then the craving rebounds, and you want more sugar! If you are one of these people who constantly craves sweets, you may want to consider how often you indulge. Think about it. We have all heard people say "I'm just not a sweets person." This is because they don't regularly eat sweets. On the contrary, those who are "regular sugar-cravers" consume more than their fair share. Simply put, the more you eat, the more you crave. The problem with sugar is not when you have an occasional sweet food, but when you eat excessive sugar. And that is easy to do as sugar is added to many processed foods, including bread, yogurt, juices, cereals and sauces.

FYI: The average American teen eats 28 teaspoons of added sugar per day. To lower the risk for heart disease, The American Heart Association recommends limiting added sugar to about 6 teaspoons per day.

Next time you pick up a candy bar, pay attention to how you feel after you eat it. How is your energy level? Are you truly satisfied or still hungry? Are you craving more? When trying to adapt to a healthy way of eating, it can be a "real eye-opener" if you just take a few minutes to observe how your body feels and the cues it is providing. So what can you do to satisfy your sweet tooth without overdoing the sugar? Have no fear! Your sugar cravings can be controlled. The key is to be mindful when choosing sweets. Have a variety of go-to sweet snacks that won't break the calorie bank. When you have a craving for sweets, sometimes you can find ways to not give in. Going for a walk or picking up a good book can take your mind off the need for a sweet. But when that fails, you need a backup plan! Here is a list of suggestion to help you stay in control while feeding your sweet tooth:

1. **Go for fruit**. The healthiest "hands-down" sweet food is fruit. If a sweet dish of pineapple, strawberries, mango, or other fruit will do the trick, this is truly the best choice. You will get a nice burst of energy but due to the fiber, your blood sugar will not drop quickly. Keeping fresh or frozen fruit always available is a great way to feed your sweet tooth and stay on track with your healthy eating routine.

2. **Keep to your meal routine.** Eat every three to five hours throughout the day will help keep your blood sugar stable and decrease your urge for the sweet stuff. Enjoying a serving of fruit with each meal will further decrease your sweet tooth.

3. **Combine your sweet with something healthy to avoid the spikes and plummets that leave you wanting more.** Maybe fresh fruit

by itself doesn't do the trick! But what if it's dipped in chocolate? YUM!! Buy a bag of chocolate chips (milk chocolate or dark–whatever your preference!) Cut up a cup of your favorite fruit. Measure out 2 tablespoons of chocolate chips (which is 130 calories) and microwave it for 30 seconds. Sit down at the table and dip the fruit into the chocolate. Or make a trail mix with 1/2 cup Multigrain Cheerios, 1 tbsp. chocolate chips and 1 tbsp chopped walnuts. Very delicious and under 220 calories!

4. **Go for the good stuff!** Choose quality over quantity. You will be more satisfied with a rich chocolate truffle or a small bar of high-quality chocolate than an average, everyday slightly-stale cookie.

5. **Feed your craving!** Enjoy what you crave, instead of denying yourself. Just try to keep to a sensible portion and eat it slowly! **Its smart to limit snacks to 200 calories.** If you feel the strong desire for a candy bar or M&Ms, go for the small size but always read the label. The small package of M&Ms is 250 calories. If you keep them in freezer, you may find that even just a small handful of frozen chocolate will make you quite happy! Try to feed your craving with something that will satisfy you so you don't continue eating. Try a small handful of nuts mixed with a tablespoon of chocolate chips. Or a granola bar with an apple or small banana.

6. **Go out and move.** When you feel a sugar craving coming on, put on your sneakers and go out for a walk. Doing something else that will relax you may take your mind off the craving. Or, if it's late at night, sip a cup of soothing chamomile tea with a teaspoon of honey to feed your sweet tooth and relax.

7. **Grab a stick of gum.** When you want something sweet, try a piece of gum. Research shows that chewing gum may help decrease your sugar craving.

10. Overindulging on any Occasion

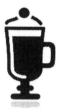

Let's face it. Everyone overindulges or overeats. Parties, vacations and holidays are celebrated every year. You have one plate of food at a party. And then you fill the plate **again**. Sinful desserts abound and beckon to you to have a taste! There are times when you have a delicious box of gourmet-style cookies sitting on your pantry shelf. You may be able to enjoy one or two during the course of a day. Other times you find yourself ready to eat the entire box. I'll say it again: **everyone indulges on occasion**. The important thing to remember is if you do overindulge (i.e., go a little overboard at a party or during the month-long winter holiday season with sweets galore everywhere or when you are home late at night watching TV), **get right back on track with your meal routine**.

Here are some suggestions to get you back on track:

1. **If you are not hungry and simply feel like gorging, stop and ask yourself why you are doing this.** Are you bored, lonely, stressed or just feeling down? It helps to know that there are many other ways to resolve these feelings without eating. Many times if you can figure out why you are eating for reasons other than hunger, you can find other ways to cope that don't revolve around food.

2. **Find a way to decrease stress without eating.** Exercise is one of the best stress relievers. Exercise can help you feel better. It improves your mood, boosts your confidence, increases your energy level, and improves your overall outlook on life. If exercise is new to you, discover what you enjoy. Attempt an exercise video, go for a power walk, participate in a group exercise class or meet with an exercise buddy at your local gym. A cup of herbal tea or picking up a good book may help you relax. Some other ways to de-stress or fill these voids include calling a friend or family member and writing down your thoughts in a journal. The point is to explore other avenues of coping. Remind yourself food is meant to nourish your body. If you are using food for other reasons or feel down regularly, you may need to talk with a friend, parent, school psychologist or your physician.

3. **Do not ignore how you are feeling.** Tell yourself that these foods are not adding any nourishment to your body. Just a lot of excess calories. If throwing out the cookies, cake or candy will keep you from devouring them, then get rid of them. Don't let overeating interfere with working towards your healthy goals of losing weight and eating well. If you do experience that feeling of self-pity that usually occurs after you've eaten one too many cookies or had more than two slices of that delicious birthday cake (you know what I mean!), stop that negativity as soon as you can. Just because you ate too much doesn't make you "bad." Eating too much does not make you a failure. Don't get down on yourself and let everything you worked for just go out the window. Be positive! Pick yourself up, practice positive self-talk, and get back on track. **Always love yourself no matter what!**

4. **You are a wonderful person**. Regardless of your body size or what you just put in your mouth, that is irrelevant! Whatever

you do, don't forget that. This is a simple, yet significant concept you must understand: **you must take care of yourself and love yourself in order to healthfully achieve your goals**. Always be kind to yourself! Choose to *not* let overeating sabotage your healthy goals of eating well and maintaining a healthy weight.

5. **Realize that everybody eats too much on certain occasions.** It's not the end of the world. When you get back on track and eat healthy, the positive benefits of practicing self-care will follow you through.

6. **Practice self-monitoring if you find it hard to get back on track.** Start to keep a daily food record. Seeing what you are eating can help motivate you to continue on with eating healthy. It can make a big difference when you see things on paper as opposed to keeping it in your head.

Tips to Help You Avoid or Limit Overindulging

1. **Read food labels.** Knowing the calorie content will help you limit your intake and stick to portion sizes.

2. **Keep a daily food and feelings journal.** Recording everything you eat, as well as the time and how you are feeling when you eat. Not only will keeping a journal help you to see what you are *really* consuming but it may help you better understand your weaknesses and timings of when you overeat. Read your journal and recognize how good you feel when you make the healthy choice.

3. **Write down your healthy goals and share them with a loved one.** Goals should serve as a constant motivator. Sharing them with a loved one will provide additional support you may need when faced with temptation.

4. **Make it easy to be healthy.** Know what foods you tend to "give-in" to and do not have these food items around. Fill your pantry with healthy foods.

5. **Find healthy alternatives to your vices.** If you love candy bars, try granola bars. If you love chips, try raw vegetables with hummus. If you love ice cream, try frozen fruit (make fresh frozen fruit sorbet) or low fat yogurt (you can stir up the yogurt and freeze it!).

6. **Eat slowly and drink lots of water.** Pace yourself and you will eat less. Fill up on water and you will get full faster.

7. **Wean yourself off sweets.** As you take sweets out of your diet and increase your intake of healthy foods such as fruits and vegetables, you will lessen the desire for these sugar-packed, low-nutrient foods.

8. **Eat every three to five hours.** Listen to your body and eat when you are hungry to maintain a constant energy level. This will help you avoid overeating.

9. **Exercise.** Exercise increases your energy, improves your metabolism, raises your confidence, enhances your mood and helps you balance your food intake.

10. **Seek professional help if you feel you need it**. Talk with your parents or school psychologist. They are there to help you.

11. **Treat yourself with a non-food reward.** When you feel you deserve a reward, try one of these: go see that movie you've been dying to see, or take a walk in the park with your dog, get tickets to that concert you've had your heart set on or purchase that beautiful dress you've been eyeing. Avoid using food as a reward.

PART 3

Tools of the Trade

Introduction

1. Weight Management

2. Nutrition Basics

3. Learn How to Cook

4. Helpful Apps for Reaching Your Health Goals

5. How to Spot a Fad Diet

6. Tips for Preventing an Eating Disorder

7. Standard Portion Sizes

8. Sample Meal Plans

9. Deliciously Healthy Meal and Snack Ideas

10. One-Week Menu

11. Healthy Shopping List

12. What's up with Vegetarian and Vegan Diets

13. "Take Away" Healthy Eating Tips

14. Finding a Registered Dietitian for Individualized Help

15. Recommended Books and Websites

16. Contact me (my blog, consultations via email)

17. Recipes

Introduction

As you should know by now, healthy eating plus exercise are the gold standards for enjoying a desired weight and a healthy life. Here are the tools, tips, apps and recipes to guide you on the path to healthy eating and living. In addition you will find important info on how to "sniff out" a fad diet as well as timely tips on preventing an eating disorder. This toolbox also incudes a sample meal plan, along with a shopping list, a one-week menu and additional meal and snack suggestions. The recipes at the end of this section were chosen because they are easy to prepare, very nutritious, won't break the calorie bank and are quite tasty as well. Hopefully they will become part of your "go-to" recipe file for many years to come! Good luck on your journey to looking and feeling great!

1. Tools of the Trade: Weight Management 101

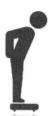

What is my healthy weight range?

Because many teens are still growing, this is not an easy question to answer. In fact, from the time you start puberty you can grow an additional ten inches or more. Girls usually stop growing in height shortly after they start their period, but boys can grow throughout their college years. In addition to gaining height, your bones and muscle mass continue to develop. Your weight will increase as your body develops, so your healthy weight range can be constantly changing until you are fully grown. To figure out your healthy weight range you need to first determine your BMI (body mass index) and then plot it on a graph to determine what percentage you are in for your age.

Visit this link to **easily figure out** your healthy weight range: http://kidshealth.org/teen/food_fitness/dieting/weight_height.html#_height.

Should I be Counting Calories?

Some people find that counting calories helps them stay on track and lose weight. Counting calories can help you eat less but you also want to make sure that you are eating healthy. **My professional advice:** count the number of servings from each food group throughout your day. By following this method you can **limit** your calories, but ensure that you are eating a variety of healthy foods. In Section 8 (Sample Meal Plans) there are two sample meal plans that are gender-specific. Each sample meal plan will tell you how many servings per day you should have from each of the six food groups. Use the one that is appropriate for you as a guide when planning your daily meals and snacks. You can also use one of the apps such as LoseIt or FitDay to keep your daily food log. However when the app tells you how many calories you have left for the day, please consider how many foods you have left from each group for your remaining meals and/or snack calories. Also, don't have less than 1500 calories per day if you are a female. And for males, don't eat less than 1800 calories per day. Adjust the calories if the LoseIt or Fitday app tells you to eat less than 1500 or 1800 calories per day. Eating too little calories will decrease your metabolism and make it harder for you to lose, as well as maintain, your weight. Become familiar with how many servings you should have daily from each food group. If you still feel hungry at the end of a meal have another serving of non-starchy vegetables or salad. Or if you have not eaten your daily fruit quota, have a fruit. Non-starchy vegetables and fruit are low in calories, rich in fiber and nutrient powerhouses. That's why they should be at least 50% of your lunch and dinner meals.

What is a "healthy weight loss"? *One pound per week* is a safe amount of weight to lose. If you lose weight quickly, it will most likely not be sustainable. Losing weight too quickly can also limit your growth potential for height. It will also decrease muscle mass. On the other hand, if you lose weight slowly, you are more likely to learn new healthy habits and stick with them. And then you will be much more likely to maintain your desired weight. That is what having a healthy meal routine and maintaining your weight is all about. Make these new skills you've learned **sustainable habits**! It takes about one month to practice a new habit and make it lasting. Focus on healthy eating and daily exercise. The weight that you lose will be the reward for taking good care of yourself!

2. Tools of the Trade: Nutrition Basics

Here's a brief overview of the basics (protein, carbohydrate and fat) plus info on key nutrients that should be included as part of your daily meal routine.

Calories

Purpose: The calories, from the food you eat, provide you with the energy, or fuel, to accomplish what you want to do. Think of calories like gasoline for your car. If your gas tank is on empty, your car won't budge. Replenish your calories throughout the day to keep your energy level high!

Protein

Purpose: Protein is required for many functions in the body. It's found in almost every part of the body, including hair, nails, skin, bones, muscle and blood. Protein synthesizes tissues needed for wound healing. Enzymes and hemoglobin, the oxygen-carrying part of blood, are also derived from protein. Antibodies, which protect against bacteria that can cause illness and/or infection, are made from proteins. It is also important for the synthesis of hormones, such as insulin, which helps to regulate blood sugar (or glucose). Although we only require approx. 20% of our daily calories from protein, we need to consume protein daily as our bodies are unable to store it. Each gram of protein provides 4 calories.

Recommendations: Females between the ages of 14 to 19 years need approximately 46 grams of protein per day. Males between the ages of 14 to 19 require approximately 52 grams of protein daily.

Food Sources: Protein is available from both animal and plant sources. Animal proteins include meat, fish, chicken, eggs, milk, cheese and yogurt. Plant proteins are found in nuts, seeds, beans, tofu, edamame, nut butter, tempeh, seitan, soymilk, vegetables and whole grains (cereal and breads).

It's easy to meet your protein quota. In fact, many Americans consume too much protein. Excess protein makes your kidneys, whose one of many roles is to remove waste products from the blood, work on overtime. It can also excrete calcium from your bones, which can lead to osteoporosis in the future. So make sure to get your daily quota, but don't over-do-it!

See how easy it is to get protein:

1 cup (8 oz.) milk or yogurt = 8 grams
1 egg = 7 grams
3 oz. chicken, fish or lean meat = 21 grams
4 oz. tofu = 10 grams
1/2 cup beans (chickpeas, black beans, etc.) = 6 grams
1 cup (8 oz.) soy milk =10 grams
2 tbsp. peanut butter = 7 grams

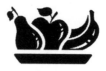

Carbohydrate

Purpose: Carbohydrate is the primary energy source for your body. Your brain must have carbohydrate to function. Plant foods, which are nutrient powerhouses, are also known as complex carbohydrates.

Recommendations: 50 to 65% of the total calories of your diet should come from carbohydrate. If you are consuming 1800 calories per day, this is approximately 270 grams of carbohydrate (or 1080 calories). For 1500 calories per day, this equals 225 grams (900 calories) of carbohydrate. Each gram of carbohydrate contains 4 calories.

Food sources: The healthiest carbohydrates are complex carbohydrates. These include fruits, non-starchy vegetables (such as broccoli, carrots, zucchini and cucumbers), whole grains (including breads, cereals, rice, pasta, barley and quinoa) and starchy vegetables (such as potatoes, butternut squash and beans). Unhealthy carbohydrates are refined carbohydrates. This group includes candy, soda, juice drinks and refined breads and cereals. Try to limit these foods as much as possible. Although they may taste good, they have little nutritional value and, therefore, not so good for you!

Fat

Purpose: Fats provide the body with an important source of energy. Fat also has many other functions including:

1. Fat helps keep you warm by providing the body with insulation.

2. Fat also cushions all of the body's organs.

3. Helps the body absorb the fat-soluble vitamins: A, E, D and K.

4. Having a small amount of fat at a meal or snack can enhance satiety (the sensation of feeling full), which can help people eat less and increase weight loss.

5. Fat is also vital for healthy skin and hair.

Recommendations: 25 to 35 % of daily calorie intake should come from fat. In a 1800 calorie meal plan, 540 calories (60 grams) should be consumed as fat. A 1500-calorie meal plan should contain 450 calories (or 50 grams) of fat. Each gram of fat provides 9 calories.

Food sources: Healthy sources: Nuts, nut butter, avocados, olives, olive oil and canola oil. Limit saturated and trans fats, which can clog your arteries and increase the risk of heart disease. Saturated fats include butter, full-fat cheese, 2% and whole milk, fatty meats (including bacon, sausage and spare ribs), coconut and palm oils. Avoid all trans fats (baked goods such as cookies, muffins and doughnuts, cracker and chips, fried foods, vegetable shortening and stick margarine). If a product label states 0 trans fats, but it contains partially hydrogenated or hydrogenated fats or shortening in the ingredient list, it does have trans fats. Leave the product on the shelf!

In addition to getting a healthy supply of calories, protein, carbohydrate and fat in your diet, you need to get your fair share of vitamins and minerals. **Below are a listing of vitamins and minerals that are important for teens to emphasize in their diets.** Try to choose foods that are good sources of these key nutrients at each of your meals and snacks. It's always better to eat healthy foods than to rely on vitamin and mineral supplements for good nutrition.

Minerals:

Iron

Purpose: Iron, as part of hemoglobin, carries oxygen from the lungs throughout the body. It is also required for the synthesis of all cells. Iron is also a part of many enzymes, which helps the body to digest foods and utilize nutrients.

Recommendations: Male teens require 11 mgs of iron per day. Female teens need 15 to 18 mgs of iron per day.

Food sources: There are two types of dietary iron: **Heme-iron** is from animal foods such as fish, shellfish, poultry and lean meat. **Non-heme iron** sources are plant foods and include beans (such as chickpeas, lentils and black beans), iron-fortified breads and cereals, and spinach. To increase the amount of iron absorbed at a meal, include a good source of Vitamin C such citrus fruit (orange, lemon, grapefruit), tomatoes, and/or broccoli.

Here is where you'll find iron:
Heme-iron sources:
3 ounces cooked lean meat: 3 mgs
3 ounces cooked turkey: 3 mgs
3 ounces cooked white meat chicken: 1 mg

Non-heme iron sources:
1 cup fortified instant oatmeal: 10 mgs
1 cup cooked soybeans (edamame): 8 mgs
1 cup cooked kidney beans: 5 mgs

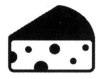

Calcium

Purpose: Builds bones and helps them stay strong. Also essential for forming teeth when you are young. Necessary for blood-clotting, heart rhythm and muscle function.

Recommendations: 1300 mgs per day for teens which equals 3 to 4 servings of high-calcium foods per day

Food sources: Calcium is widely abundant in dairy products, such as milk, yogurt and cheese. In addition, you can also find this important bone-builder in calcium-fortified soy and almond milk, sardines and canned salmon (you must eat the soft bones to get the calcium!), tofu that is made with calcium sulfate (please check ingredient label) and leafy greens, such as kale.

Here's a variety of choices to get your calcium from:		
Soymilk, calcium-fortified	1 cup	300 mgs
Skim milk	1 cup	300 mgs
Almond milk, calcium-fortified	1 cup	300 mgs
Cheddar cheese	1.5 oz.	307 mgs
Mozzarella, part-skim	1.5 oz.	333 mgs
Tofu, firm (made with calcium sulfate)	4 oz.	250 mgs
Sardines, canned in oil, with bones	3 oz.	325 mgs
Kale, raw or cooked	1 cup	90 mgs
Turnip greens, boiled	1/2 cup	99 mgs
Bok Choy), raw	1 cup	74 mgs

Potassium

Purpose: This important mineral is essential for optimal heart and muscle function. Potassium also helps maintain fluid balance and the building of strong bones. Potassium-rich foods also helps regulate blood pressure. Making sure you eat foods high in potassium now may help you keep your blood pressure in control as you get older.

Recommendations: For teens ages 14 to 18, you need 4700 mgs of potassium daily.

Food sources: Fruits and vegetables, beans, whole grains, dairy, lean meats and fish.
Check out these rich-potassium food sources:

1 cup white beans:	1,189 mgs
1 cup cooked spinach:	839 mgs
1 cup nonfat yogurt:	580 mgs
1 small banana:	470 mgs
1 medium orange:	300 mgs
1 cup broccoli:	457 mgs
1 cup cantaloupe:	430 mgs

Vitamins:
Vitamin D

Purpose: Vitamin D has been shown to be vital to good health for so many reasons:
1. It's essential for absorption of calcium to help maximize bone growth and strength. A low intake can lead to soft bones and osteoporosis later in life.
2. A deficiency of Vitamin D has been linked to a variety of health conditions including breast and colon cancer, heart disease and depression.

Recommendations: Approximately 600 IU for teens ages 13- 19 years old.

Food sources: The body makes vitamin D when exposed to sunlight. It can store extra vitamin D for later use. Try to get some sunshine everyday. Food sources include fortified-dairy products, including milk and yogurt plus fortified soymilk. Fatty fish, such as salmon and tuna, are also rich sources of vitamin D.

Get your Vitamin D quota here:

3 ounces salmon, cooked	447 IU
3 ounces tuna fish, canned in water, drained	154 IU
1 cup milk, vitamin-D fortified	120 IU
1 cup yogurt, fortified with 20% DV	80 IU
1 large egg (D is in yolk only)	41 IU
1 cup fortified cereal with 10% DV	40 IU

3. Tools of the Trade: Learn How to Cook

Taking the time to learn how to cook will provide you an abundance of delicious benefits. When you cook you have the ability to make healthy meals plus have food taste the way **you** want. You can create your own healthy meals that you enjoy. Learning how to chop, dice, saute', grill and roast foods are culinary techniques that will put wonderful meals on your table. Although going out to eat is enjoyable for a variety of reasons, including someone else prepares the food and you don't have to clean the dishes(!), you don't always know exactly what your eating. If you rely often on restaurants and take-out, you may take in too many calories (think bread basket and large portions!), in addition to excessive salt, fat, and quite often, too much sugar. Unless you order your meal to be grilled or broiled or cooked simply without sauces or oil, the food may not be prepared as healthy as you think. Being able to prepare your own meals at home will help you get more nutrition on your plate. It also comes in handy when you have friends over and you can serve them a great meal that you prepared. **Read my lips:** nothing beats home cooking! Read the ten tips which sum up why it 's so important to know how to cook.

10 Reasons Why You Should Learn How to Cook

1. **Health:** You can eat healthier. You buy the ingredients, so you know what is going on your plate! You can prepare more nutritious foods and avoid pre-packaged, processed items.

2. **Quality:** You can control what is going into your food. You can limit (or completely avoid) the amount and type of fat as well as salt, sugar and harmful additives that goes into your meal.

3. **Cost:** You will save money! The average lunch meal in a restaurant is $10.00 (not including tax and tip). You can make a delicious lunch or dinner meal for $2.50 or less!

4. **Taste:** Home-cooked meals taste better! Learning to cook can help you achieve delicious flavors by learning what works and what doesn't work in the kitchen. You can take a handful of simple ingredients and–voila!–turn them into delicious meals.

5. **Social:** You can have guests over and serve them your tasty creations. It's a great way to entertain friends and showcase your talents! Plus you can also entertain at home without "breaking the bank!"

6. **Weight management:** Cooking at home will help you manage your weight. You can eat less calories because you will know exactly how much you are eating. You won't have to "guesstimate" like you do when you eat in a restaurant.

7. **Culture:** You can broaden your horizons by cooking various ethnic dishes. Experiencing different cuisines can give the feeling of traveling to exotic places. When you experience different tastes from other regions of the world, you are also learning about other cultures through food. Cooking is a learning experience!

8. **Convenience:** When we cook for ourselves we can make our meals more convenient by preparing additional foods in advance. For example, you can make a large salad or roasted vegetables so you have leftovers for a couple days or make a soup or chili and freeze it for an easy dinner. Thus you won't have to rely on unhealthy take-out and fast food when time is tight.

9. **Independence-** Learning to cook can give you a great sense of freedom and independence. Knowing you are able to cook is a wonderful skill to have. And you will have the personal satisfaction of knowing that you are can care for yourself by preparing nourishing meals.

10. **Life Enrichment-**Learning how to cook has so many wonderful benefits, besides making delicious meals. Getting involved in cooking can become a hobby or passion that enhances you life. Taking cooking classes, developing recipes you try out on family or friends or traveling to exotic places to experience local cuisine can bring much pleasure along with adventure. Many people have taken their love of food and cooking and turned it into their dream job.

Here is a list of awesome cookbooks that will help you enhance your cooking skills. At the very end of this section are an array of healthy simple-to-prepare recipes that you should find are good basic dishes for you to start with.

Recommended Cookbooks

1. Mark Bittman, "How to Cook Everything—The Basics," (Wiley 2012)

2. Irma S. Rombauer, Marion Rombauer Becker and Ethan Becker, "Joy of Cooking," (Simon and Schuster 2006)

3. Jackie Newgent, RD "The Big Green Cookbook," (Wiley 2009)

4. Vacarello, Liz and Mindy Hermann,RD, "The 400 Calorie Fixes" (Rodale 2011)

5. Dawn Jackson Blatner, "The Flexitarian Diet," (McGraw Hill 2008)

4. Tools of the Trade: Helpful Apps for Good Health

Here is a list of "top-notch" apps that can help you reach your health and weight goals. Use them to make your life easier, healthier and tastier! From apps for making the healthiest food choices and cooking tasty dishes to workout routines that get you toned and fit, these apps have it all!

Weight Loss Apps

LoseIt (free) iPhone or www.loseit.com This simple and fun app helps you to get going with your healthy meal routine plus stay on track. LoseIt has a daily calorie intake budget, lets you set your personal goals plus keeps tabs on your exercise. You can also add new foods and exercises to the program. In addition, there is a free barcode scanner to evaluate food products and progress charts to help encourage users. My personal favorite!

MyFitnessPal (free) compatible with iPhone and Android www.myfitnesspal.com Has the largest food database of all apps along with a vast exercise list. This fast and easy diet app is free for both the iPhone and Android. It has a large food database with millions of different foods, brands and restaurants. Also documents your food and water intake and exercise plus has barcode scanner.

80 Bites ($0.99) iPhone Like a pedometer for your mouth. Helps improve you're eating behavior. Slows down your eating by counting your bites! Become aware of what you eat and how fast you eat it!

Teen BMI (free) iPhone. It shows you what your healthy BMI (body mass index) range is. BMI is based on your age, gender, weight and height.

Exercise Apps

Nike Training Club (free) iPhone
Get lean and in shape with the free app for the iPhone. This is your own personal trainer 24/7. There are over 60 custom workouts, over 90 multi-directional drills for strength, cardio, and core training, as well as specific regimens from professional athletes. You can chose workouts that fit your criteria and the app has audio guidance to keep you on track and working hard.

Track Your Steps: iSteps ($0.99) iPhone Works like a pedometer! Counts your steps, distance, average speed and calories burned. You can wear it on your waist (with a clip) or carry it in your hand as you walk. Great and easy way to get healthy and promote exercise. So press "start" and get moving!

Couch-to-5K ($0.99) helps you train to become a runner. Spend just 20 to 30 minutes three times per week for nine weeks and you'll be running over three miles at a clip! Provides you with support so you can meet your goals.

Recipe Apps

SparkRecipes: HealthyRecipes (free) for Apple products. Eat healthy and save money! It simplifies 'cooking like a chef" with over 190,000 recipes to search from. Browse the search engine by course, ethnicity, prep time and more. Includes nutrition analysis for each dish plus cooking videos to improve your kitchen skills.

Good Food Healthy Recipes (BBC Worldwide) ($0.99 for Apple products) 175 healthy recipes with nutrition info to keep you eating well throughout the year. Recipes for meals, snacks and desserts, plus videos to help you perfect your cooking skills.

Cooking Light–Quick and Healthy Menu Maker ($3.99) iPhone and iPad. Create your own menu along with a nutrition calculator that works as you create it. Over 300 entrees, sides, and desserts. Allows you to save and share your favorite menus and recipes via email, Facebook and twitter.

Nutrition info Apps

CalorieKing (free) iPhone Contains over 70,000 foods and menus for 260 restaurants and fast food chains. Can easily compare foods for nutrition info. Will help you stay on track with healthy eating and meeting your weight loss goals. Truly one of the best! Highly recommend!!

FastFood Calories ($0.99) iPhone Includes nutrition info from over 100 fast food and chain restaurants. With this app you can easily make smarter choices when dining out.

CalorieCounter (free for Apple products). Will count your daily calorie intake. Contains barcode scanner which can add food to you intake. Large food database.

Grocery Shopping Apps

Fooducate (free for Apple products) Become more knowledgeable about what you are purchasing in the grocery store. Scan the barcodes and choose the healthiest groceries in the stores. Large database of different foods. Compare products and receive healthier alternatives. This app is like a personal dietitian in your pocket!

ShopWell (Free) for iPhone. Input you health goals and this app will help you make the right choices in the grocery store. Eat more healthy foods and steer clear of the foods you should avoid. Scan a food's barcode and see if it is right for you based on your goals.

Motivational Apps

App Resolutions ($0.99) for iPhone. Unique for making resolutions at New Years and throughout the year. Select from a list or create your custom resolution. Features a "Tip of the Day" to motivate you to meet your weight and exercise goals.

MyLilCoach for iPhone **and MyLilCoach2** for iPhone4 ($1.99) It's a reminder, pedometer and coach all rolled up in one app! Helps you follow a healthy lifestyle: eat mindfully, drink water, exercise and reduce stress. MyLilCoach will remind you throughout the day, even when the app is closed. A terrific multi-purpose app!

Track Your Entire Life: The Carrot (free) www.thecarrot.com Not only does it help you track food and exercise but you can also track your sleep habits, mood, weight, and more! Calculates your daily calorie intake as well as calories you burn from different types of workouts. Great motivational app.

5. Tools of the Trade: How to Spot a Fad Diet

Fad diets don't work. Besides being unhealthy, they don't provide sustainable long-term results. The smartest way to safely lose weight is to make healthy food choices and exercise regularly with no gimmicks and no foods to exclude. While there is no set approach to identifying a fad diet, many have the following characteristics:

- Recommendations that promise a quick fix.
- Dire warnings of dangers from a single product or regimen.
- Claims that sound too good to be true.
- Simplistic conclusions drawn from a complex study.
- Recommendations based on a single study or testimonials.
- Dramatic statements that are refuted by reputable scientific organizations.
- Lists of 'good' and 'bad' foods.
- Recommendations made to help sell a product.
- Recommendations based on studies published without review by other researchers.
- Recommendations from studies that ignore differences among individuals or groups.
- Eliminating 1 or more of the 5 food groups (dairy and non-dairy alternatives, proteins, fruits/vegetables, whole grains/starchy vegetables and fats).

6. Tools of the Trade: Tips for Preventing an Eating Disorder

*Learn all you can about anorexia nervosa, bulimia nervosa, and binge eating disorder.

 *Genuine awareness will help you avoid judgmental or mistaken attitudes about food, weight, body shape, and eating disorders.

*Discourage the idea that a particular diet, weight, or body size will automatically lead to happiness and fulfillment.

*Choose to challenge the false belief that thinness and weight loss are great, while body fat and weight gain are horrible or indicate laziness, worthlessness, or immorality.

*Avoid categorizing foods as "good/safe" vs. "bad/dangerous." Remember, we all need to eat a balanced variety of foods.

*Decide to avoid judging others and yourself on the basis of body weight or shape. Turn off the voices in your head that tell you that a person's body weight says anything about their character, personality, or value as a person.

*Become a critical viewer of the media and its messages about self-esteem and body image. Talk back to the television when you hear a comment or see an image that promotes thinness at all costs. Rip out (or better yet, write to the editor) advertisements or articles in your magazines that make you feel bad about your body shape or size.

*If you think someone has an eating disorder, express your concerns in a forthright, caring manner. Gently but firmly encourage the person to seek trained professional help.

*Decide to avoid judging others and yourself on the basis of body weight or shape. Turn off the voices in your head that tell you that a person's body weight says anything about their character, personality, or value as a person.

*Avoid conveying an attitude that says, "I will like you better if you lose weight, or don't eat so much, etc."

*Be a model of healthy self-esteem and body image. Recognize that others pay attention and learn from the way you talk about yourself and your body. Choose to talk about yourself with respect and appreciation. Choose to value yourself based on your goals, accomplishments, talents, and character. Avoid letting the way you feel about your body weight and shape determine the course of your day. Embrace the natural diversity of human bodies and celebrate your body's unique shape and size.

*Support local and national nonprofit eating disorders organizations — like the National Eating Disorders Association — by volunteering your time or giving a tax-deductible donation.

Don't Weigh Your Self-Esteem, It's What's Inside That Counts!

Copyright 2005 National Eating Disorder Association
www.NationalEatingDisorders.org
Information and Referral Helpline 800-931-2237

7. Tools of the Trade: Standard Portion Sizes*

Food	Portion	Looks Like
Fresh fruit (such as an apple or orange)	1 piece (=1 cup fruit)	Tennis ball
Dried fruit	1/4 cup	Golf ball
Berries	1 cup	Baseball
Meat, poultry or fish	3 ounces	1 deck of cards
Peanut butter	2 tablespoons	Walnut in the shell
Nuts	2 tablespoons	1 golf ball
Hard cheese	1 1/2 ounces	Six dice
Cold cereal, dry	1 cup is 1 grain	Baseball serving)
Legumes (beans, lentils)	1 cup, cooked	Baseball
Rice or pasta	1 cup is 3 grain	Baseball servings)
Popcorn (no oil)	3 cups (=1 grain)	Three baseballs
Pancake or waffle	1	Compact disc

Salad dressing	1 tablespoon	1/2 shot glass
Oil (such as olive)	1 teaspoon	Standard cap of 16 oz. water bottle
Margarine, butter or mayonnaise	1 teaspoon	Standard post stamp

*Adapted from (c) 2005 The Portion Teller by Lisa R. Young, PhD, RD

8. Tools of the Trade: Sample Healthy Meal Plans

Introduction to the Meal Plan

The meal plans featured here are to be used as a guide in planning your daily meals. Use this meal template to help you plan what to eat for breakfast, lunch, dinner and snacks. The meal plan will also tell you how many daily servings to have from each food group. If you still feel hungry at the end of a meal, have another serving of vegetables or salad. As stated before, snacks are at your discretion. If you are hungry or know you will be exercising within the next couple of hours, have a snack. If you aren't hungry, wait until your next meal to eat. Try to eat every three to five hours. If you don't eat regularly, you may find that you get excessively hungry and then eat too much at the next meal. **Always be mindful** of what and when you are eating!

For females: The following meal plan will help guide you in deciding how to plan your meals. This meal plan is approximately 1500 calories which may be appropriate for teenage girls who would like to lose weight and are not very active. If you are active (exercising for one hour at least four times per week) increase the calories to 1800 per day. For 1800 calories add these **extras**: add 2 bread/starch servings, 1 fruit and 2 proteins.

Sample Healthy Meal Plan-1500 calories (for females)
<u>Daily exchanges per day</u>

Dairy/Soy	2 servings (nonfat) = skim, soy, almond milk or yogurt
Fruit	3 servings
Vegetables	2+ servings
Proteins	7 ounces
Grain/Starch 6 servings	
Fat	4 tsp (mono=best—avocado, nut butter, olive or canola oil)

<u>Sample menu</u>
Breakfast
1 cup high fiber cereal or 2 waffles or whole grain English muffin 1 cup skim or 1% milk or calcium-fortified soy or almond milk
1 oz. low fat cheese or 1 egg or 10 nuts or ½ cup 1% cottage cheese
1 fruit

Lunch
3 oz. lean protein (fish or poultry) or 6 oz. tofu or 2 tbsp. peanut butter or 1 cup beans
2 slices whole grain bread or 1 sandwich thin or 1 cup beans
1 tsp olive oil /vinegar or squeeze of fresh lemon
salad or raw/cooked vegetables
water

Snack
1 fruit + 1 granola bar or 10 nuts or 1 cup nonfat yogurt or 1 cup cereal + 1 cup skim/soy/almond milk

Dinner
3 oz. chicken, fish or lean meat or 5 oz. tofu or 1 cup beans
large salad and steamed or raw vegetables
2 tbsp. low fat salad dressing or 1 tbsp olive oil/vinegar/lemon
2/3 cup pasta or 1 medium potato or 1 ear corn plus 1 slice bread

Snack 1 fruit or 1 cup nonfat yogurt or 1 granola bar or 1 cup dry cereal

For males: The 1800 calorie meal plan is appropriate for you if you are not very active. If you are active (exercise for one hour four times per week), increase meal plan to 2100 calories per day. To achieve 2100 calories: add 2 bread/starch, 1 fruit and 2 proteins.

Sample Healthy Meal Plan-1800 calories (for males)
Daily exchanges per day

Dairy/Soy	2 servings (nonfat) = skim milk, soy milk, plain yogurt
Fruit	3 servings
Vegetables	2+ servings
Proteins	9 ounces
Grain/Starch	8 servings
Fat	4 tsp (monounsaturated are best—Olive, canola or peanut)

Sample menu
Breakfast
1 cup high fiber cereal or granola bar or 2 waffles or 2 slices ww toast
1 cup skim or 1% milk, soy or almond milk

1 oz. low fat cheese or 1 egg or 10 nuts or ½ cup 1% cottage cheese
1 fruit

Lunch
4 oz. lean protein (fish, poultry or lean meat) or 6 oz. tofu or 2 tbsp. PB
2 slices whole grain bread or 1 cup beans or 1 slice bread + 1 other starch
1 tsp olive oil
salad or raw vegetables
water

Snack
1 fruit + 1 granola bar or 10 nuts or 1 cup nonfat yogurt + 1 fruit or 1 cup cereal w/milk

Dinner
4 oz. chicken, fish, meat or 5 oz. tofu or 1 cup beans such as chickpeas
large salad
steamed or raw vegetables
2 tbsp. low fat salad dressing or 1 tbsp olive oil/vinegar/lemon
2/3 cup pasta or 1 medium potato or 1 ear corn plus 1 slice bread

Snack
1 fruit + 1 granola bar OR 1 cup cereal + 1 cup skim or alternative milk

9. Deliciously Healthy and Filling Meal and Snack Ideas

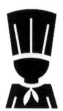

Here are a variety of healthy quick-and-easy suggestions for breakfast, lunch, dinner and snacks. Use these ideas to help you stay on track with your meal routine.

Breakfast:
*1 cup cereal such as Multigrain Cheerios or Barbara's Cinnamon Puffins + 1 cup skim or soy milk + 1 small banana + 10 almonds
*1/2 cup low fat cottage cheese mixed with 1 cup blueberries
+ 1 with 1 tablespoon peanut butter + 1 Thomas's Whole Grain Bagel Thin
*1 Arnold's Whole Grain Sandwich Thin + 2 tbsp. natural peanut butter + 1 small banana
*Make a parfait: 1 cup nonfat Greek yogurt + 1 cup cereal
+ 1/2 cup sliced strawberries (add 1 teaspoon of sugar if not sweet enough) + 1 tbsp nuts
Breakfast sandwich: 1 Arnold's Whole Grain Sandwich Thin
+ 1 scrambled egg + 1 slice 2% cheese (such as Cabot's or Baby Bel) + tomato slices + 1 orange
If you are in a hurry: grab 1 granola bar + 1 cup nonfat yogurt and 1 apple

Lunch:

*1 Arnold's Whole Grain Sandwich Thin + 2 tbsp hummus + 1/4 avocado slices + 2 tomato slices + side of carrot sticks and cucumber slices. Finish the meal with 1 apple, banana, peach or nectarine.

*Spinach salad: 1 bowl (2 cups) of baby spinach. Add 3 ounces grilled chicken + 1/2 cup small white beans + 1 tbsp sliced almonds or chopped walnuts + 1 orange, peeled and sliced. Dressing: 2 tbsp. lite vinaigrette.

*100 calorie whole wheat wrap with baby greens + shredded carrots + sliced tomato with 2 ounces low fat mozzarella cheese. Finish the meal with an apple or orange.

*Turkey sandwich: 2 slices whole grain bread + 3 ounces turkey breast + 1/4 avocado, sliced + side of raw carrot sticks + 1 orange or banana.

*Veggie burger: 1 Arnold's Whole Grain Sandwich Thin + 1 veggie burger (Amy's, Morningstar Farms, Gardenburger or Dr. Praeger's are all good choices) + 1/4 sliced avocado or 1 slice low fat cheese. Complete the meal with 1 cup of fresh strawberries or blueberries.

Dinner:

*Pasta with summer vegetables: Start with 1 cup whole wheat pasta, cooked. Sautee' 2 tsp. olive oil + 2 cloves sliced garlic. Add 2 cups chopped broccoli and cauliflower plus 1 cup sliced grape tomatoes, sliced in half. When veggies are done, add pasta to pan and mix together. Complete the meal with 1 orange or small pink grapefruit. Save any (!) leftovers for another meal.

*3 ounces grilled salmon on a bed of sauteed peppers, onions and mushrooms. Add a salad (2 cups) of mixed greens with 1 tbsp. lite vinaigrette. Complete the meal with a cup of strawberries.

*3 ounces grilled chicken + 1/2 cup brown rice + 2 cups roasted veggies (zucchini + red peppers + onions). Roast veggies with 2 tsp. olive oil and pinch of salt at 400 degrees till slightly browned. Make a salad with baby spinach + 1/4 avocado, sliced and fresh orange slices. **Timesaver:** You can make extra roasted veggies for the next day! Make a sandwich (for lunch) with the roasted veggies + 2 tbsp. hummus or 2 ounces low fat cheese or toss with 1 cup whole grain pasta for dinner.

*2 cups homemade vegetable soup or 1 can such as Amy's + large salad (3 cups baby spinach or mixed greens + 1 tbsp chopped nuts + 1 chopped cucumber + 1 chopped carrot + 1/2 cup grapes (cut in half). Dressing: 2 tbsp lite vinaigrette.

Snacks:

*1 granola bar + 1 fresh fruit

*1/2 cup 1% cottage cheese + 1 cup blueberries

*Smoothie: 1 cup plain nonfat yogurt or skim or soymilk + 1 serving of fresh or frozen fruit. Fill blender with ice to top. Blend and enjoy!

*1 cup whole grain cereal (such as Multigrain Cheerios, Kashi Heart to Heart or Barbara's Cinnamon Puffins + 1 cup skim, soy or almond milk

*1 can Amy's soup, such as Minestrone or Vegetable Barley (look for soups that have 100 calories or less and at least 4 grams of fiber **per serving**

*100-calorie bag of popcorn and 1 fruit

*4 tbsp. hummus with cucumber slices and/or carrots, celery sticks, red pepper

10. Tools of the Trade: One-Week Menu

Use this menu as a guide if you need some help planning your meals and snacks.

	Breakfast	Lunch	Snack	Dinner	Snack
Sunday	1 cup Cheerios 1 c.skim/soy milk 1 small banana 10 almonds Coffee/tea	peanut butter and sliced apple sandwich (2 T. PB) on whole grain bread 2 raw carrots 1 orange Water or green tea	1 Kashi TLC granola bar	3 ounces grilled chicken 1 cup sauteed broccoli salad: romaine, red onion, tomatoes, cucmbers, 1/2 cup chickpeas 1 t olive oil w/ fresh lemon Water or seltzer	1 pear 1 cheese stick
Monday	1 whole wheat English muffin w/1 ounce cheese and sl. tomato 1 orange 1 c. soy milk or nonfat plain yogurt-coffee or tea	Hummus sandwich (2 tbsp. hummus, cucmber/tomato slices on ww bread or pita 1 apple w ater or green tea	1 small banana 10 walnut halves or almonds	4 ounces grilled salmon with lemon and oregano Salad: tomatoes, fresh parsley, red onion and 1/2 c. chickpeas 1 cup cooked zucchini water or green tea	1 apple 1 Kashi TLC granola bar

	Breakfast	**Lunch**	**Snack**	**Dinner**	**Snack**
Tuesday	2 wholegrain waffles (Nutrigrain or Kashi) 1 cup blueberries 10 almonds 1c.skim/soy coffee or tea	tuna salad sw on whole grain bread: 3 oz. tuna w/1 tbsp light mayo and chopped celery raw carrots and cucumber 1 peach water/seltzer	1 cup non-fat Greek yogurt 1/2 cup sliced strawberries	3 ounces chicken sauteed with grape tomatoes and basil1 ear corn salad: baby spinach w/ 5 sliced strawberries and 1 tbsp chopped nuts 2 t olive oil/vinegar water or seltzer	1 Kashi TLC granola bar or 100 calorie bag of popcorn
Wednesday	1 cup Barbara's Cinnamon Puffins 1 small banana 1 hard boiled egg 1 c.skim/soy milk coffee/tea with 1 tablespoon milk	Cheese and tomato s/w (2 oz. cheese, tomato and basil on whole grain) 1 orange water or green tea	1 apple and 10 almonds	1 cup multi-grain pasta w/2 cups sauteed broccoli and mushrooms-salad: lettuce, tomato, red pepper 2 t olive oil + lemon water or tea	1 orange and 1 cheese stick

	Breakfast	**Lunch**	**Snack**	**Dinner**	**Snack**
Thursday	1 cup Kashi Heart to Heart 10 almonds 1 small banana 1 cup skim or soy milk coffee/tea	Egg salad s/w: 1 egg plus 1 t. mayo on ww bread Raw carrots and cucumbers 1 plum water/green tea	1 Kashi TLC granola bar	3 oz. grilled fish 1 cup quinoa w/sauteed zucchini and onion salad: romaine and tomatoes 2 t olive oil w/ fresh lemon water or seltzer	1 pear and 10 almonds
Friday	1 scrambled egg and 1 oz cheese on ww English muffin 1 orange coffee/tea	Almond butter (2 T.) and banana slices on 2 sl ww toast Raw carrots and celery water/green tea	1 cup non-fat Greek yogurt 1 apple	Grilled portobello mushroom burger or turkey burger with 1/4 sliced avocado and tomato on 2 sl.ww bread- Salad: Baby spinach, grape tomatoes and 1 T. chopped walnuts 2 t. olive oil/ vinegar	1 Kashi TLC granola bar and 1 fruit

	Breakfast	**Lunch**	**Snack**	**Dinner**	**Snack**
Saturday	1 scrambled egg and 1 oz cheese on ww English muffin 2 sl. vegetarian bacon 1 orange coffee/tea	Sandwich: grilled veggies with 1 oz. cheese Salad: halved grape tomatoes, red onion, fresh parsley with 1 t. olive oil and fresh lemon Grapes (17 small)	1 Kashi TLC granola bar	1 slice pizza w/ large salad or 3 ounces grilled chicken 2 cups sauteed broccoli salad with 1/2 cup small white beans and tomatoes	1 cup fresh fruit salad

11. Tools of the Trade: Healthy Shopping List

These foods are some of the best in the grocery store. Try to include them as part of your daily diet. In addition to managing your weight, eating well can help prevent disease and enhance the quality of your life. Foods with fiber are strongly encouraged as they not only help prevent disease, but also aid in weight management by keeping you full.

Cereals: Purchase cereals that have at least 3 grams dietary fiber and not more than 6 grams of sugar per serving. Good brands = Kashi Heart to Heart, Kashi Autumn Harvest, Barbara's Cinnamon Puffins, Barbara's Shredded Spoonfuls and Cheerios (Plain or Multigrain). Limit the serving to 1 cup. Whole grain cereal (1 cup) is also good for a snack.

Bread: Whole grains are best. Look for the word "whole" at the beginning of the ingredient list. Whole grain breads should have at least 2 grams of dietary fiber per serving. To save on calories, try the lite whole grain breads. Arnold's Whole Grain Sandwich Thins or Thomas's Whole Grain Bagel Thins are great for sandwiches.

Healthy granola bars: Kashi TLC, Lara Bars, Clif Bars and Kind Bars are all good choices. Look for bars that are 200 calories or less, contain at least 4 grams of protein and 4 grams of fiber per serving. Sugar should be 6 grams or less per bar. Limit bars to 2 per day. If you are in a rush have 2 bars for breakfast or lunch (but don't make this a regular thing!).

Starchy vegetables/Grains: These complex carbohydrates include beans (such as kidney, chickpeas, lentils, black beans and cannellini beans), sweet and white potatoes, acorn and butternut squash, brown rice, quinoa, barley, whole wheat couscous, amaranth, buckwheat (or kasha), whole grain pasta, peas and corn. Because beans have the highest fiber content (8 grams per 1/2 cup), aim to have **at least** 1/2 cup (4 ounces) three times per week.

Soups: "Health Valley" and "Amy's"– great-tasting vegetarian soups; moderate in sodium/ high in fiber, broth-based vegetable and bean soups are the healthiest choices. These soups are great as part of a meal or for a snack. Or make your own healthy vegetable soup and freeze it in batches.

Best margarines: Tub margarines are best. Should contain 0 grams trans fats. Good brands = Take Control, Benecol, Smart Balance and Olivio.

Best oils/fat— Monounsaturated and omega-3 fats. Mono = olive oil, olives, canola oil, nuts, nut butters and avocados. Omega-3 = fatty fish (wild salmon, tuna, mackerel, herring and sardines, bluefish), nuts and ground flax and/or chia seed.

Heart-healthy fish: wild salmon, tuna, mackerel, herring, sardines, bluefish—aim for 6 oz. per week. Fatty fish also contain omega-3 fats.

Milk: Calcium-fortified soy or almond milk and organic skim or 1% milk.

Yogurt: Good brands = Phage, Chobani, Stonyfield, Horizon, Colombo and Dannon. These yogurts contain live cultures. The healthiest is nonfat plain. Add your own fresh fruit for a sweet kick. If you need more sweetness, add one teaspoon sugar or stevia and stir.

Cheese: low fat is best (3 grams fat per ounce). Good choices = Cabot's, Baby Bel and Laughing Cow. Use whole fat cheese (9 grams fat/ounce) in moderation (limit to 2 ounces per day).

Proteins: include more vegetarian proteins in your diet such as tofu, beans, hummus and nuts/ nut butters. Limit red meat (beef, lamb, pork and veal) to three times per week (3 ounces cooked per meal) or less. Eat more veggie burgers, beans, tofu, fish, eggs and chicken instead of red meat.

Fruits: have at least 2 servings per day. Fresh whole fruit is best. Limit or avoid juice as it doesn't contain any fiber and is very concentrated in sugar. And it won't fill you. Water is always the better choice!

Vegetables: aim for a minimum of 3 cups or more per day. Fresh or frozen (without sauce) is best. Fill at least 1/2 of your plate with vegetables!

Snacks: limit to 200 calories per snack. Good choices=Kashi TLC granola bars (140 calories each) or Kind bars, 100 calorie bags of popcorn, fresh fruit and 1 ounce protein such as low fat cheese or 10 nuts or 8 oz. nonfat yogurt. A cup of cereal and nonfat milk or a can of vegetable soup are also good options.

Healthy sweeteners: Stevia is a healthy sweetener and has 0 calories. Use sugar, fruit juice and honey in moderation.
1 packet sugar has 16 calories and 4 grams carbohydrate.

Best beverage: water, seltzer, coffee, green and white tea, herb teas. Drink at least 8 cups daily to stay hydrated. Use 1 packet of stevia or sugar if you want your beverage sweetened. If you want to have a diet soda, limit to 1 per day. Clear diet sodas, such as Diet 7-Up, are a better choice as colas contain phosphates, which can leach calcium from bone.

12. Tools of the Trade: Vegetarian vs. Vegan Diets

With increasing knowledge regarding the health benefits of consuming plant-based foods and documentaries galore advocating less consumption of animal products, it is no wonder vegetarian and vegan diets have surged as popular ways to eat. Teens may choose to follow either diet for a variety of reasons: animal rights, protecting the planet, parental preferences, religious beliefs and/or improved health are just a few. Followed correctly, each can offer several health benefits such as lowering the risk for heart disease, Type 2 diabetes and many types of cancer. However, if animal products are not substituted appropriately, the risk for running deficient in certain nutrients, including protein, vitamins and minerals is raised. So proceed with care. Both diets can be very healthy ways to eat if done right.

If you are interested in following either diet you should be fond of vegetables, whole grains and non-meat alternatives such as tofu, nuts and beans as these will all serve as the basis for many of your meals. It is essential you take the time to educate yourself on how to properly follow these diets. If well-thought out and well-planned, nutrition deficiencies can be avoided, health benefits gained and you will be fit and fueled. To guarantee you follow a well-balanced vegetarian or vegan diet, you should meet with a Registered Dietitian (RD) to receive expert nutritional guidance.

Let's look at these two diets and see how they differ:

Vegetarian diets can be sub-divided into a few different categories. **True vegetarians** (also known as **lacto-ovo vegetarians**) avoid all meat, fish and poultry but do consume eggs and dairy products. **Lacto-vegetarians** eat dairy products but avoid eggs, meat, fish and poultry, and **ovo-vegetarians** eat eggs but avoid dairy, meat, fish and poultry. Similarly, **"flexitarian" and "semi-vegetarian,"** which are basically the same, describe a diet that consists largely of vegetarian items with the occasional meat, fish or poultry source thrown into the mix. Vegetarians who also eat fish are known as **pescatarians**.

True vegetarians typically obtain protein from dairy (milk, yogurt and cheese), eggs and soy products. Tempeh, a texturized protein made from soybeans, brown rice, millet and barley, and seitan, made from wheat gluten (a protein found in wheat), are two meat alternatives many vegetarians also include in their diet. With a wide variety of complete protein sources available, the vegetarian diet is easy to follow with little risk for deficiency.

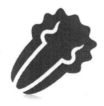

Compared to the vegetarian diet, **vegan diets** require more planning to ensure that adequate protein, vitamins and minerals are consumed. Those following a true vegan diet avoid all foods from animal sources. Meat, fish, poultry, eggs, dairy and butter are avoided. Many vegans also avoid honey. With fewer options for protein, plant-based proteins, such as soy products (tofu and soy milk), tempeh, beans, nuts, legumes, seitan, vegetables and whole grains become the staples.

Teens who want to follow a vegan diet need to make sure that they get sufficient nutrients, such as protein and calcium to fuel growth. To ensure adequate protein is consumed, a variety of these plant-protein foods mentioned above should be consumed regularly at meals. As stated before, a RD should be consulted to ensure that the diet is well planned. Because vitamin B-12 is found only in animal products, vegans need to supplement their diet with this vitamin. The vegan may seek out fortified food sources, such as soymilk fortified with vitamin B-12, to obtain this vitamin or simply take in the form of a pill supplement. Since dairy products are not consumed, calcium can also become an issue so appropriate food alternatives, such as calcium-fortified tofu, soy or almond milk and dark green leafy vegetables, need to be included in the diet daily. If nutritional needs for calcium can't be obtained through food alone, a calcium supplement should be taken. Teens that follow a vegan diet also need to pay special attention to getting enough vitamin D, calcium, iron, zinc and iodine. In order to obtain the health benefits of either a vegetarian or vegan diet, the diets need to be followed properly.

Differences between Vegetarian and Vegan Diets

Diet	Vegetarian	Vegan
Foods included	Milk, cheese, butter, eggs, grains, tofu, seitan, tempeh, nuts, beans, fruits, vegetables,	Tofu, seitan, tempeh, nuts, beans, whole grain breads and cereals, fortified-soy and almond milk, fruits and vegetables.
Foods avoided	Meat, fish, chicken	Milk, cheese, butter, meat, fish. chicken, eggs, dairy (some vegans also avoid honey)
Nutrients which may be lacking	Vegetarians should be able to easily meet all of their nutrient needs if they make healthy food choices.	Vegans need to take a vitamin B12 supplement. If food sources of vitamin D, iron, calcium, zinc and iodine don't meet nutritional needs, a supplement may be needed.

13. Tools of the Trade: Take-Away Healthy Eating Tips

1. Start every morning with breakfast.

2. Eat at least three meals (breakfast, lunch and dinner) every day. Snacks are optional.

3. Always stick to your meal routine.

4. Eat mindfully. Count slowly to 20 with each bite. Use a small plate.

5. Always keep a couple healthy granola bars on hand in case you feel hungry. Limit to two/day.

6. Fill up on non-starchy vegetables, such as broccoli, cauliflower, tomatoes, cucumbers and carrots, at lunch and dinner. At least 1/2 of your plate should be vegetables.

7. Fresh or frozen fruit is the best dessert.

8. Drink water throughout the day: two cups per meal and at least one per snack.

9. Eat every three to five hours.

10. Keep a daily food log to keep yourself on track with your meal routine.

11. Exercise every day. Walking your dog counts! Turn on your pedometer in the morning when you wake up and aim for 10,000 steps each day.

12. Love yourself no matter what. You are wonderful no matter what your weight is. As you practice self-care and take good care of yourself, you will reach your healthy weight!

14. Tools of the Trade: Finding a Registered Dietitian for Individual Help and Guidance

To find a Registered Dietitian/Nutritionist (RD) in your area, please go to the website: www.eatright.org (which is the website of The Academy of Nutrition and Dietetics). Click on "Find a Registered Dietitian" in the upper right-hand corner. Type in your zip code and find an RD in your area. You can also see the specific areas that the RD specializes in. You may want to choose someone with experience working with teens and weight management. Please feel free to email me (eatwellrd@yahoo.com) if you are not successful in finding an RD to help you reach your health and weight loss goals. I will do my best to find someone you can work with.

15. Tools of the Trade: Recommended Books and Websites

Books

Nutrition Information Books
1. Brian Wansink, PhD, "Mindless Eating" (Bantam 2006)
2. Dr. Lisa Young, PhD, RD, "Portion Teller" (Broadway 2005).
3. Roberta Duyff, MS, RD, "Food and Nutrition Guide" (3rd Ed., Wiley 2006)
4. Nancy Clark, "Nancy Clark's Sports Nutrition Guidebook" (Human Kinetics, 2008).
5. Elisa Zied, MS, RD, "Nutrition at Your Fingertips" (Alpha 2009)
6. Evelyn Tribole, MS, RD and Elyse Resch, MS, RD, "Intuitive Eating" (St. Martin's Press 2012)
7. Bonnie Taub-Dix, MA, RD, CDN, "Read It Before You Eat It" (Plume 2010)

Cookbooks
1. Mark Bittman, "How to Cook Everything—The Basics" (Wiley 2012)
2. Irma S. Rombauer, Marion Rombauer Becker and Ethan Becker, "Joy of Cooking" (Simon and Schuster 2006)
3. Jackie Newgent, RD "The Big Green Cookbook" (Wiley 2009)
4. Vacarello, Liz and Mindy Hermann,RD, "The 400 Calorie Fixes" (Rodale 2011)
5. Dawn Jackson Blatner, RD, "The Flexitarian Diet" (McGraw Hill 2008)

Websites

1. **Bodimojo** (www.bodimojo.com) This amazing site personalizes health info just for teens. Great resource for updates on body image, nutrition, emotional life, dating, exercise and more. Highly recommend!

2. **The 2008 Physical Activity Guidelines for Americans**, from the U.S. Department of Health and Human Services. http://www.health.gov/PAGuidelines is where you can learn about the benefits of physical activity. Provides general information on physical activity including how often you should be active and which activities are best for you.

3. **The President's Council on Physical Fitness and Sports** http://www.fitness.gov . Provides regular updates on the Council's activities as well as resources on how to get involved in its programs.

4. **Girl's Health** http://www.girlshealth.gov, developed by the Office on Women's Health, Excellent resource for female teens on physical activity, nutrition, stress reduction, and more.

5. **USDA's Team Nutrition** website http://www.fns.usda.gov/tn . Focuses on the role nutritious school meals, nutrition education, and a health-promoting school environment play in helping students learn to enjoy healthy eating and physical activity.

6. **Bone Health Campaign** http://www.bestbonesforever.gov is a sponsored by the Office of Women's Health. For girls and their friends to grow stronger together and stay strong forever.

7. **National Diabetes Education Program for teens**. http://ndep.nih.gov/teens/index.aspx, This website offers publications and resources on how teens can prevent and manage diabetes.

8. http://hin.nhlbi.nih.gov/portion/keep.htm is a quiz from the **National Heart, Lung, and Blood Institute** that tests your knowledge of how food portion sizes have changed during the last 20 years.

9. **CDC's Division of Nutrition and Physical Activity**. http://www. cdc.gov/nccdphp/dnpa/physical/index.htm. Provides recommendations on how to get started on a fitness program with links to websites that offer health information for teens.

16. Tools of the Trade: Contact me

If you would like to be in contact with me for either a nutrition consultation or if you have any nutrition-related questions, you can connect with me at:

Email: eatwellrd@yahoo.com

My websites: www.lisastollmanrd.com

www.teeneatingmanifesto.com

My blog: www.eatingmanifesto.com

Follow me on twitter: twitter.com/eatwellrd

Follow me on facebook: www.facebook.com/lisa.stollman

17. Tools of the Trade: Healthy Recipes

Here is a collection of healthy recipes that are simple-to-make and high in nutrient content! If you have never cooked before, now is the time to experiment and find recipes you love and can share with your family and friends. Look for recipes online and put together a collection of your favorites!

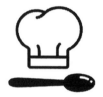

Beverages
Fruit Smoothie
Watermelon Cooler
Pineapple Smoothie

Snacks/Dips
Kale chips (delicious and healthy alternative to potato chips)
Trail Mix
Hummus
Black Bean Salsa
Guacamole

Soups
Italian Bean and Vegetable Soup
Black Bean Soup
Asian Vegetable Soup

Salads
Mediterranean Salad
Mixed Greens with Roasted Red Peppers, White Beans and Feta
Red Oak Leaf Salad with Raspberries and Walnuts
Health Slaw
Quinoa Summer Salad

Vegetables
Baked Sweet Potato Fries
Roasted Cauliflower (any vegetable can be substituted in this recipe!)

Sandwiches
Egg Salad Sandwich
Peanut Butter and Green Apple Toast
Hummus Sandwich (Veggie Delight)
Portobello Mushroom Burger
Greek Pizza Muffin

Entrees
Vegetarian Chili
Mediterranean Chicken Couscous
Bow Ties with Tomato and Feta
Roasted Tofu

Desserts
Fruit Sundae
Fruit Sorbet
Fruit Salad

BEVERAGES

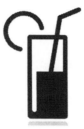

Fresh Fruit Smoothie

Yield: 1 serving

Ingredients
1 small banana or 1 cup berries
1 cup skim, soy or almond milk
Ice

Put first two ingredients in blender.
Fill rest of blender with ice.
Blend until frothy. Enjoy!

Nutrition info:
 Serving size: 1 serving
 Calories: 150
 Protein: 3 grams
 Carbohydrate: 24 grams
 Fiber: 2 grams
 Sugar: 24 grams
 Fat: 1.5 grams
 Sodium: 120 mgs

Watermelon Cooler
Yield: 2
Ingredients:
2 cups chilled watermelon cubes

Put watermelon cubes in blender. Blend a couple minutes till frothy.
Pour into glass and enjoy. Great with lunch or dinner!

Nutrition info:
Serving size:1 cup
Calories: 50
Protein: 0 grams
Carbohydrate: 12 grams
Sugar: 12 grams
Fiber: .6 grams
Fat: 0 grams
Sodium: 3 mgs

Pineapple Smoothie (Courtesy of Dana White, RD)
Servings: 1
Ingredients:
½ medium banana, sliced and frozen (freeze ahead of time)
½ cup frozen pineapple chunks
¼ cup nonfat Greek-style yogurt, plain
½ cup orange juice
¼ cup water

Directions: Combine ingredients in a blender. Blend until smooth.

Nutrition info:
Serving size: 2 cups
Calories: 176

Protein: 7 grams
Carbohydrate: 38 grams
Fiber: 3 grams
Sugar: 38 grams
Total Fat: 0.5 gram
Sodium: 25 milligrams

SNACKS/DIPS

Kale Chips (delicious and healthy alternative to potato chips)
Yield: 4 servings

Ingredients:
4 cups kale
1 tbsp. olive oil
1 teaspoon salt
Optional seasonings if desired (cumin, red pepper flakes, curry)

1. Preheat oven to 375 degrees F. Rinse the kale leaves and dry them. Cut the kale leaves off of the center stalk.
2. Cut the leaves into two-inch pieces. Put the cut kale in a bowl. Add in the olive oil and mix with the kale.
3. Add salt and any other seasonings you desire and toss well.
4. Arrange the kale in a single layer on a nonstick baking sheet or a Pyrex dish.
5. Bake for about 20 minutes or until the kale looks crispy and is turning brown on the edges.
6. Put the kale chips in a bowl and let cool for 5 minutes before eating. Kale chips will stay crispy for two to three days in an airtight container.

Nutrition info:
Serving size: 1 cup
Calories: 65
Protein: 3 grams

Fat: 4 grams
Carbohydrate: 8 grams
Sugar: 0 grams
Dietary fiber: 2 grams
Sodium: 425 mgs

SUGAR AND SPICE TRAIL MIX

This is a perfect snack. Keep this in a re-sealable plastic bag in your backpack or gym bag and you'll have energy to enjoy your day! It's sweet, but not too sweet.

Yield: 10 servings
Ingredients:
3 cups oat squares cereal
3 cups mini-pretzels, salted or salt-free, as desired
2 tablespoons tub margarine, melted
1 tablespoon packed brown sugar
1/2 teaspoon cinnamon
1 cup dried fruit bits or raisins
1. Preheat oven to 325F.

1. In a large re-sealable plastic bag or plastic container with a cover, combine the oat squares and pretzels.
2. In a small microwavable bowl, melt the margarine, and add the brown sugar and cinnamon. Mix well. Pour over the cereal mixture.
3. Seal the bag or container and shake gently until the mixture is well coated.
4. Transfer to a baking sheet.
5. Bake uncovered for 15 to 20 minutes, stirring once or twice.
6. Let cool. Then add the dried fruit.
7. Store in an airtight container or smaller single-serving bags.

Nutrition Info:
Serving size: 1/2 cup (4 oz.)
Calories per serving: 200
Carbohydrate: 40 grams
Protein: 5 grams
Fat 2 grams

Recipe courtesy "Nancy Clark's Sports Nutrition Guidebook," 4th Edition, Human Kinetics Publisher by Nancy Clark, RD and the American Heart Association (www.deliciousdecisions.com)

DIPS/SPREADS

Hummus
Yield: 16 servings

Ingredients:
I (15.5 ounce) can chickpeas
1 tbsp tahini (sesame seed butter) or olive oil
Optional for adding different flavors: 1 tbsp. fresh lemon juice or 1 tsp. cumin, red pepper or chopped garlic. Experiment as you please!

Put chickpeas and tahini or olive oil in blender. Add lemon juice or herbs as desired.
Blend in blender until all ingredients are mixed thoroughly. You may need to stop the blender and push ingredients down with spoon as mixture will be quite thick.
Serve with raw cut-up vegetables or as sandwich spread with cucumbers and tomato slices on whole grain bread.

Nutrition info:
  Serving size: 2 tablespoons
  Calories: 40
  Protein: 1 gram
  Carbohydrate: 4.5 grams
  Dietary fiber: 2 grams
  Sugar: .5 grams
  Fat: 1 gram
  Sodium: 33 mgs

Black Bean Salsa   (adapted from Nutrition Action Newsletter (**www.cspi.org)**

Great as a dip with raw vegetables, as a taco filling or with grilled chicken or fish.
Yield: 4 Servings

Ingredients:
1 (16 ounce can) black beans, (rinsed and drained)
1 avocado, chopped into small pieces
1 small red onion, chopped
2 tbsp fresh cilantro leaves, chopped

Combine all ingredients in a bowl.
Season with the juice of a half a lime and 1/4 tsp. salt.

Nutrition info:
Serving size: 1/4 of recipe (approx. 3/4 of a cup)
Calories: 193
Protein: 9 grams
Carbohydrate: 29 grams
Sugar: 0 grams
Dietary Fiber: 5 grams

Fat: 7.5 grams
Sodium: 346 mgs

Guacamole
Yield: 4 servings

Ingredients:
1 avocado, chopped into 1 inch pieces
1 large tomato, chopped into small pieces
1 cucumber, peeled and chopped into small pieces
1 yellow medium onion, chopped.
1/2 teaspoon salt
Pepper

In medium size bowl add first four ingredients and mix all together.
Season with salt and pepper.
Serve with sliced cucumbers and yellow/red peppers.

Nutrition info:
Serving size: 1/4 of recipe
Calories: 97
Protein: 2.55 grams
Carbohydrate: 11.4 grams
Sugar: 0 grams
Dietary fiber: 5.45
Fat: 7.8 grams
Sodium: 292

SOUPS

Italian Bean and Vegetable Soup

Yield: 8 servings

Ingredients
1 tablespoon olive oil
1 cup chopped onion
1 cup sliced carrot
1/2 cup chopped green bell pepper
2 garlic cloves, crushed
1 (32-ounce) box vegetable broth
1 (28-ounce) can crushed tomatoes
1 (15-ounce) can cannellini (small, white) beans, rinsed and drained
1 (15-ounce) can red kidney beans, rinsed and drained
1 1/2 teaspoons dried Italian seasoning
1/4 teaspoon black pepper
6 ounces uncooked whole wheat rotini pasta
1/4 cup grated fresh Parmesan cheese

Preparation
1. Heat oil in a large Dutch oven coated with cooking spray over medium-high heat. Add onion and next 3 ingredients; sauté until vegetables are crisp-tender.
2. Add beef broth and next 6 ingredients; bring to a boil. Cover, reduce heat, and simmer 20 minutes, stirring occasionally.

3. Add pasta to vegetable mixture. Cover and cook 10 to 15 minutes or until pasta is tender.

4. Ladle soup into individual bowls; top each serving with 1 tablespoon cheese.

Nutrition info:
> Serving size: 1 1/4 cups
> Calories: 232
> Protein: 10.8g
> Fat: 4.5g
> Carbohydrate: 36.2g
> Fiber: 4.2g
> Cholesterol: 5 mgs
> Sodium: 497 mgs

Black Bean Soup
Yield: 4 servings.

Ingredients:
4 cups vegetable or chicken broth.
1 (15-ounce) can black beans
3 chopped tomatoes
1 (1.4 ounce) can green chili peppers
2 tablespoons olive oil
4 garlic cloves, minced
1 tablespoon cumin
Fresh cilantro (optional)

Sautee 1 chopped onion, 1 tablespoon cumin, and 4 minced garlic cloves in 2 tablespoons olive oil.

Add 4 cups vegetable or chicken broth, 3 chopped tomatoes, one 15-ounce can black beans, and one 1.4-ounce can diced green chili peppers.

Bring to a boil, cover and simmer 5 minutes.

Add 2 tablespoons snipped fresh cilantro.

Nutrition info:
 Serving size: 1 1/2 cups
 Calories: 245
 Protein: 10 grams
 Carbohydrate: 34 grams
 Fiber: 8 grams
 Sugar: 0 grams
 Fat: 11 grams
 Sodium: 929 mgs

Asian Vegetable Soup
Yield: 4 servings

Ingredients:
1 tablespoon canola oil
1 garlic clove, minced
3 scallions
3 medium stalks bok choy or celery
2 medium carrots
15 snow peas
4 cups vegetable broth
2 teaspoon lite soy sauce
1 teaspoon ground ginger

1. In medium soup pot, heal oil over medium heat.
2. Remove end and tips of scallions and chop into small pieces. Add scallion and garlic to pan and sautee'.
3. Remove 1 inch from stalk end of celery or Bok Choy and slice stalk and leaves into thin slices. Add to pot and cook until soft.
4. Cut snow peas diagonally into thirds and add to pot.
5. Peel and chop carrots and add to pot.
6. Add soy sauce and vegetable broth and cook over medium heat.
7. Lower heat to simmer and add ginger.
8. Cook until carrots have softened.

Nutrition info:
Serving size: 8 ounces (1 cup)
Calories: 65
Protein: 3 grams
Fat: 3 grams
Carbohydrate: 5 grams
Sugar: 2 grams
Fiber: 3 grams
Sodium: 228 mgs

SALADS

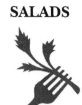

Mediterranean Salad

Yield: 4 servings

Ingredients:
1 16 ounce can chickpeas or white cannellini beans
1 cup grape tomatoes, halved
1 small red onion, chopped
1 small bunch flat Italian parsley, chopped
1 tbsp. olive oil
2 tsp. red wine vinegar or fresh lemon juice
1 teaspoon salt
Pepper to taste

Directions:
1. Rinse and drain chickpeas and place in salad bowl.
2. Add tomatoes, red onion and parsley.
3. Stir together olive oil, vinegar, salt and pepper.
4. Pour over salad and serve.

Nutrition info:
    Serving size: 1 cup
    Calories: 153
    Protein: 8 grams
    Fat: 4 grams

Carbohydrate: 27 grams
Fiber: 6 grams
Sugar: 0 grams
Sodium: 344 mgs

Health Slaw

Yield: 4 servings

Ingredients
1 cup shredded carrots (about 2 large carrots)
1 cup shredded red cabbage
2 tablespoons balsamic vinegar
1 tablespoon olive oil
1 tablespoon honey
1/4 teaspoon salt

Put first two ingredients in large bowl. Mix next four ingredients together and pour over salad. Toss salad to combine all ingredients. Cover and refrigerate until ready to serve.

Nutrition info:
Serving size: 1/2 cup
Calories: 70
Protein: .7 grams
Carbohydrate: 10 grams
Fiber: 2 grams
Sugar: 4 grams
Fat: 3.5 grams
Sodium: 174 mgs

Mixed Greens with Roasted Peppers, White Beans, Red Onion and Feta (Courtesy of Dana White, RD)

Yield: 6 servings

Ingredients:
8 ounces (about 8 cups) pre-washed baby greens
½ small red onion, sliced thin
1 cup roasted red peppers (packed in water), cut into thin strips
½ 16-ounce can (about 3/4 cup) small white beans, drained
½ cup crumbled feta cheese
¼ cup extra-virgin olive oil
Ground black pepper
1½ tablespoons fresh lemon juice

Instructions:
Place salad greens, red onion, roasted peppers, white beans, and feta in a large salad bowl.
Toss with olive oil and a sprinkling of ground black pepper.
Add lemon juice; toss to coat. Taste adding more lemon juice if necessary. Serve.

Nutrition info:
    Serving size: approx. 1 1/2 cups
    Calories: 180
    Protein: 5.6 grams
    Fat: 14 grams
    Carbohydrate: 11 grams
    Fiber: 3 grams
    Sugar: 0 grams
    Sodium: 319 mgs

Red Oak Leaf Salad with Raspberries and Walnuts (Courtesy of Sharon Palmer, RD)

Yield: 6 servings

Ingredients:
2 c. washed, torn red oak leaf lettuce
1/2 c. mozzarella cheese, shredded
1/2 c. peeled, chopped cucumbers
1 c. fresh raspberries, cleaned and drained
1/2 c. walnuts, chopped
2 tbsp. olive oil
1 tbsp. red wine vinegar

Toss lettuce, cheese, and cucumbers in bowl. Place on individual salad plates, or in salad mixing bowl. Toss olive oil and red wine vinegar together and toss into salad very lightly. Top the salad with raspberries and walnuts.

Nutrition info:
    Serving size: 1 cup
    Calories: 2oo
    Protein: 7.8 grams
    Carbohydrate: 5.6 grams
    Fiber: 3 grams
    Sugar: 1.5 grams
    Fat: 16 grams
    Sodium: 69 mgs

Quinoa Summer Salad

Yield: 4 servings

Ingredients:
1 cup water
1/2 cup uncooked quinoa
3/4 cup fresh parsley leaves
1/2 cup thinly sliced celery
1 cup chopped cucumber
1/2 cup thinly sliced green onions
1 cup red grapes, sliced in half
3 tablespoons fresh lemon juice
1 tablespoon olive oil
1 tablespoon honey
1/4 teaspoon salt
1/4 teaspoon black pepper
1/4 cup raw cashews or walnuts, chopped

Bring water and quinoa to a boil in a medium saucepan. Cover, reduce heat, and simmer 20 minutes or until liquid is absorbed. Spoon into a bowl; fluff with a fork. Add parsley, celery, onions, cucumbers, grapes and nuts.
Whisk together lemon juice, olive oil, honey, salt, and black pepper. Add to quinoa mixture and toss well.

Nutrition info
 Serving size: 1 cup
 Calories: 238
 Protein: 5.9 grams
 Carbohydrate: 35.1 grams
 Fiber: 3.6 grams
 Fat: 8.6 grams
 Sodium: 172 mgs

VEGETABLES

Roasted Cauliflower

Yield: Serves 4

Ingredients:
1 head of cauliflower
2-3 cloves of garlic, peeled and coarsely minced
1 tablespoon olive oil
1/2 teaspoon salt
2 tablespoons Parmesan cheese (optional)

1. Preheat oven to 400°F. Cut cauliflower into florets and put in a single layer in an ovenproof baking dish. Toss in the garlic. Drizzle with olive oil. Sprinkle with salt.

2. Place casserole in the oven, uncovered, for 25-30 minutes, or until the top is lightly brown. Test with a fork for desired doneness. Fork should easily pierce the cauliflower. Remove from oven and sprinkle with Parmesan cheese (optional). Serve immediately. **Note:** You can substitute almost any vegetable for the cauliflower. Roasted vegetables are delicious! Great also as a snack or in a sandwich with hummus or cheese.

Nutrition info:
    Serving size: 1 cup
    Calories: 60
    Protein: 2 grams
    Carbohydrate: 5 grams

Fiber: 3 grams
Sugar: 0 grams
Fat: 4 grams
Sodium: 290 mgs

Baked Sweet Potato Fries
Yield: 4 servings

Ingredients:
2 medium sweet potatoes (cut lengthwise into 1/3 inch strips on each side)
1 tablespoon olive oil
1 teaspoon ground cumin
1/2 teaspoon chili powder
1/2 teaspoon salt
1/2 teaspoon garlic powder

Directions
Preheat oven to 450F.
Combine all ingredients in a small mixing bowl. Mix to evenly coat potato strips.
Place potato strips on cookie sheet. Allow space between each strip for even cooking.
Bake for 15 minutes (or until potatoes are crispy) turning strips every 5 minutes or as needed.

Nutrition info:
Serving size: 1/4 of recipe
Calories 118
Protein 1 gram
Fat: 4 grams
Carbohydrates: 16 grams

Fiber: 2 grams
Sugar: 5 grams
Sodium: 300 mgs

SANDWICHES

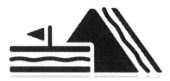

Egg Salad Sandwich

Yield: 2 sandwiches

Ingredients:
2 hard-boiled eggs, chopped
1 celery stalk, chopped
1 tablespoon mayonnaise
1 tsp. Dijon mustard (optional)
1 medium tomato, sliced thin
4 slices whole grain toast

Mix all ingredients in large bowl.
Serve on two slices whole grain toast with fresh tomato slices. Can also be served as a scoop of egg salad on top of a mixed green salad.

Nutrition info:
　　Serving size = 1 sandwich
　　Calories: 270
　　Protein: 6.3 grams
　　Fat: 11.1 grams
　　Carbohydrate: 14.7 grams
　　Fiber: 6 grams
　　Sugar: 0 grams
　　Sodium: 284 mgs

Greek Pizza Muffin (Courtesy of Barbie Cervino, MS, RD, CDN, New York

Yield: 1 serving

Ingredients:
1 whole grain English muffin
1 oz low-fat feta cheese
1 tablespoon hummus
3-4 cherry tomatoes

1. Slice cherry tomatoes.
2. Toast English muffin until desired consistency.
3. While it's still warm spread hummus on both end and sprinkle feta cheese and sliced tomatoes on top.

Nutrition info:
 Calories: 200
 Protein: 14 grams
 Carbohydrate: 35 grams
 Fiber: 6 grams
 Sugar: 0 grams
 Fat: 6.5 grams
 Sodium: 500 mgs

This make a delicious breakfast paired with a fresh fruit. As a lunch, enjoy with a side salad and a fresh fruit.

Peanut Butter & Green Apple Toast (Courtesy of Dana White, RD)

Yield: 1 serving
 Great for breakfast or snack

Ingredients:

1 slice whole grain bread, toasted

1 tablespoon natural peanut butter (creamy or crunchy)

1/2 green apple, thinly sliced

1 teaspoon honey

Directions:

Spread peanut butter on toasted bread.

Top with apple slices and a drizzle of honey.

Nutrition Info:

Serving size: 1 serving

Calories: 211

Protein: 8 grams

Total Fat: 9 grams

Carbohydrate: 24 grams

Fiber: 5 grams

Sugar: 4 grams

Sodium: 207 milligrams

Portobello Mushroom Burger

Yield: 2 servings

Ingredients:

2 large portobello mushrooms

1 tbsp. balsamic vinegar

1 tbsp. olive oil

1/4 teaspoon salt

2 whole wheat sandwich thins

Directions:

Wash mushroom caps. Pat dry. Scrape out gills with spoon, if desired.

Combine vinegar, olive oil and salt in shallow dish. Add mushrooms and turn to coat. If you have time, let mushrooms marinate for one hour (this is optional)

Remove mushrooms from marinade.

Sautee' mushrooms over medium heat 3 to 4 minutes on each side. Serve mushroom on sandwich thin with a slice of avocado or low fat cheese (optional). Add a salad and fresh fruit to complete the meal.

Nutrition info
> Serving size = 1/2 recipe
> Calories: 139
> Protein: 5.4 grams
> Fat: 2.4 grams
> Carbohydrate: 27 grams
> Fiber: 7 grams
> Sugar: 0 grams
> Sodium: 461 mgs

Hummus Sandwich

Yield: 1 sandwich

Ingredients:

2 tbsp. hummus

4 cucumber slices

2 slices tomato

2 slices avocado

1 whole grain sandwich thin

Spread hummus on one slice bread. Layer cucumber, tomato and avocado slices on top of hummus. Cover with slice of bread. Slice in half. Add a serving of fresh fruit, raw veggies or a fresh fruit smoothie. Enjoy! (This is my fave sandwich!)

Nutrition info:
> Serving size: 1 sandwich
> Calories: 235
> Protein: 4 grams
> Fat: 8.5 grams
> Carbohydrate: 20 grams
> Fiber: 6 grams
> Sugar: 0 grams
> Sodium: 270 mgs

ENTREES

Vegetarian Chili *(adapted from Cooking Light, November 1998)*

Yield: 5 servings

Ingredients:
1 tablespoon olive oil
2 cups chopped onion
3/4 cup chopped red bell pepper
3/4 cup chopped green bell pepper
1 garlic clove, minced
1 tablespoon chili powder
1 teaspoon dried Italian seasoning
1 (15-ounce) can Cannellini beans, rinsed and drained
1 (15-ounce) can tomato sauce
1 (15-ounce) can kidney beans, rinsed and drained
1 (15-ounce) can black beans, rinsed and drained
1 (14.5-ounce) can no-salt-added diced tomatoes, undrained
5 teaspoons grated Parmesan cheese (optional)

Directions:
1. Put one tablespoon olive oil into large pot and cook over medium-high heat.
2. Add onion and peppers, and sauté 10 minutes or until tender.
3. Add garlic; sauté 30 seconds.
4. Add chili powder and next 6 ingredients (chili powder through tomatoes).
5. Bring to a boil. Cover, reduce heat, and simmer 10 minutes or until thoroughly heated.
6. Ladle into soup bowls; sprinkle with cheese.

Nutrition info:
Serving size: 1 1/2-cups chili and 1 teaspoon cheese
Calories: 281
Protein: 17g
Fat: 2.1g
Carbohydrate: 53.2 grams
Sugar: 0 grams
Fiber: 9.5 grams
Sodium: 948 mgs

Mediterranean Chicken Couscous

Yield: 8 servings

Ingredients:
1 1/4 cups chicken or vegetable broth
1 (5.6-ounce) package whole wheat couscous
3 cups chopped cooked chicken (about 1 rotisserie chicken)
1 tbsp. dried basil
1 pint grape tomatoes, halved
1 1/2 tablespoons fresh lemon juice
1/4 teaspoon pepper

1. Heat broth on the stove until broth begins to boil. Place couscous in a large bowl, and stir in broth mixture. Cover and let stand 5 minutes.
2. Fluff couscous with a fork; stir in chicken and next 4 ingredients. Serve warm or cold.

Nutrition info:
    Serving size: 1 cup
    Amount per serving
    Calories: 212
    Protein: 21 g
    Carbohydrate: 17 g
    Fiber: 3 g
    Fat: 7 g
    Sodium: 455 mg

Bow Ties with Tomato and Feta

Yield: 4 servings

Ingredients:
6 ounces uncooked whole grain farfalle (bow tie pasta) or rotini
3 cups grape tomatoes, halved
1/3 cup thinly sliced fresh basil leaves
2 tablespoons balsamic vinegar
1 teaspoon Dijon mustard
2 cloves chopped garlic
1/4 teaspoon freshly ground black pepper
4 teaspoons olive oil
1 (4-ounce) package crumbled reduced-fat feta cheese

Preparation
1. Cook pasta according to package directions, omitting salt and fat.
2. Drain. Combine cooked pasta, tomatoes and basil in a large bowl.
3. While pasta cooks, combine vinegar and next 6 ingredients (through pepper) in a small bowl, stirring with a whisk.
4. Gradually add oil to vinegar mixture, stirring constantly with a whisk. Drizzle dressing over pasta.
5. Toss well to combine dressing with pasta. Add cheese and toss again.

Nutrition info:
    Serving size: 2 cups
    Calories: 320
    Protein: 14g
    Carbohydrate: 45.6g
    Fiber: 3.4g
    Fat: 9.9g
    Sodium: 400 mg

Roasted Tofu (Courtesy of Dana White, RD NY, NY)

Yield: 4 servings

Ingredients:
1 package extra firm tofu
2 tablespoons canola oil
2 teaspoons rice vinegar
2 teaspoons honey
2 teaspoons soy sauce
1 teaspoon sesame oil
1 teaspoon chili sauce (such as Siracha)

Directions:
1. Slice tofu into domino sized pieces (½ inch thick and 2 inches long).
2. Place pieces in a bowl lined with paper towels and refrigerate for 15-20 minutes to remove excess water.
3. Preheat oven to 425°F.
4. In a large bowl whisk canola oil, vinegar, honey, soy sauce, sesame oil and chili sauce.
5. Add tofu and gently toss to coat.
6. Transfer to a sheet pan and bake for 20-25 minutes (turning once) until golden brown.
7. Delicious with roasted vegetables and salad.

Nutrition info:
    Serving size: 4 ounces or 1/4 of recipe
    Calories: 105
    Protein: 10 grams
    Total Fat: 5 grams
    Carbohydrate: 4 grams
    Fiber: 1 gram
    Sugar: 8 grams
    Sodium: 172 milligrams

DESSERTS

Fruit Sundae
Yield: 2 servings
1 banana, sliced
1 cup blueberries
1 orange, peeled and cut into half-rounds
1 cup nonfat vanilla yogurt

Combine the first three ingredients in a large bowl.
Spoon 1/2 of fruit mixture into individual dessert bowls. Top each bowl with 1/2 cup yogurt.

Nutrition info:
> Serving size: 1/2 of recipe
> Calories: 203
> Protein: 6 grams
> Fat: 0 grams
> Carbohydrate: 47 grams
> Fiber: 5 grams
> Sugar: 33 grams
> Sodium: 70 mgs

Fresh Fruit Sorbet
Yield: 2 servings

Ingredients:
2 cups frozen fruit (your choice!)

Blend in blender till smooth. Divide into two bowls, serve immediately and enjoy!

Nutrition info:
    Serving size: 1 cup
    Calories: approx. 100
    Protein: 1 gram
    Fat: 0 grams
    Carbohydrate: 30 grams
    Fiber: 3 grams
    Sodium: 0 mgs

Fruit Salad with Honey dressing

Yield: 8 servings

Ingredients
2 tablespoons lemon juice
2 tablespoons honey
1 cantaloupe, seeded and cubed (about 3 cups)
1 pineapple, cored and cubed (about 4 cups)
1 cup blueberries
4 medium nectarines, sliced (about 2 cups)

In a small bowl, whisk together lemon juice and honey until blended.
Combine cantaloupe, pineapple, blueberries and nectarines in a large bowl. Chill until ready to serve. Just before serving, toss fruit with dressing and stir gently to coat. Serve cold.

Nutrition info:
    Serving size: 1 1/4 cups
    Calories: 107
    Protein: 2 grams
    Carbohydrate: 27 grams
    Fiber: 3 grams
    Sugar: 21.8 grams
    Fat: 0 grams
    Sodium: 2 mgs

References

1) Duyff, Roberta Larson, **The American Dietetic Association: Complete Food and Nutrition Guide**, (Wiley 2006).

2) Pennington, Jean A.T., **Bowes and Church's Food Values of Portions Commonly Used**," (19th Edition, J.B. Lippincott Company 2005).

3) **Evidence Analysis Library: Pediatric Overweight Evidence Analysis Project** Academy of Nutrition and Dietetics (formerly American Dietetic Association), 2009.

4) **KidsHealth.org** (for info on teens and exercise)

5) Mullen, Mary Catherine and Shield, Jodie, Childhood and **Adolescent Overweight: The Health Professional's Guide to Identification, Prevention and Treatment**, The American Dietetic Association, 2004.

6) Taub-Dix, Bonnie, **Read It Before You Eat It**, (Plume 2010)

7) Wansink, Brian, **"Mindless Eating,"** (Bantam 2006)

8) Zied, Elisa, **Nutrition At Your Fingertips**, (Alpha Books 2009)

9) **2010 Dietary Guidelines for Americans**, www.health.gov

10) **Food and Drug Administration** (www.fda.gov)

11) **Office of Dietary Suplements-National Institutes of Health** (http://ods.od.nih.gov)

12) **The American Heart Association** (www.heart.org)

13) **Increased food intake and changes in metabolic hormones in response to chronic sleep restriction alternated with short periods of sleep allowance** Am. J. Physiol. Regul. Integr. Comp. Physiol. January 1, 2012 302:R112-R117

14) **Sleep curtailment is accompanied by increased intake of calories from snacks** Am J Clin Nutr January 1, 2009 89:126-133

15) **Childhood Sleep Time and Long-Term Risk for Obesity: A 32-Year Prospective Birth Cohort Study** Pediatrics November 1, 2008 122:955-960

Made in the USA
Lexington, KY
15 July 2015